the sleep doctor's Diet Plan

LOSE WEIGHT THROUGH BETTER SLEEP

MICHAEL BREUS, PhD, DABSM

WITH DEBRA FULGHUM BRUCE, PhD

FOREWORD BY ARIANNA HUFFINGTON

RODALE.

This book is intended as a reference volume only, not as a medical manual.
The information given here is designed to help you make informed decisions about
your health. It is not intended as a substitute for any treatment that may have been prescribed
by your doctor. If you suspect that you have a medical problem, we urge you to seek
competent medical help.

Mention of specific companies, organizations, or authorities in this book does not imply
endorsement by the author or publisher, nor does mention of specific companies,
organizations, or authorities imply that they endorse this book, its author, or the publisher.

Internet addresses and telephone numbers given in this book were accurate
at the time it went to press.

© 2011 by Mindworks, Inc.
Recipes © Rodale Inc.

All rights reserved. No part of this publication may be reproduced or transmitted in any form
or by any means, electronic or mechanical, including photocopying, recording, or any other
information storage and retrieval system, without the written permission of the publisher.

Rodale books may be purchased for business or promotional use or for special sales.
For information, please write to:
Special Markets Department,
Rodale Inc., 733 Third Avenue,
New York, NY 10017

Printed in the United States of America
Rodale Inc. makes every effort to use acid-free ⊗, recycled paper ♺.

Book design by Joanna Williams
Illustration on page 140 by Karen Kuchar

Library of Congress Cataloging-in-Publication Data

Breus, Michael.
   The sleep doctor's diet plan : lose weight through better sleep / Michael Breus and Debra
Fulgham Bruce ; foreword by Arianna Huffington.
      p.   cm.
   Includes index.
   ISBN 978-1-60961-133-0 hardcover
   1. Sleep—Health aspects. 2. Weight loss—Popular works. I. Bruce, Debra Fulghum,
1951- II. Title.
RA786.B75 2011
613.7'94—dc22   2011009798

Distributed to the trade by Macmillan

2 4 6 8 10 9 7 5 3 1 hardcover

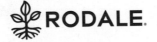

We inspire and enable people to improve their lives and the world around them.
www.rodalebooks.com

This book is dedicated to everyone
who has ever been on a diet
and wondered why it didn't work.

The time, energy, and effort I put into this book
is dedicated to my wife Lauren even though she sleeps
with the TV, cat, and Chihuahua in our bed;
and my wonderful children Mini Coop,
the best son in the whole world,
and Carson, who always reminds me that
she is my girl and full of awesomeness.
Remember, everything you do, you do better
with a good night's sleep.

Contents

Foreword by Arianna Huffington ix

Acknowledgments xiii

Introduction xv

Part I:

The Science of Sleep Meets the Science of Weight Loss

1 The Sleep/Weight Connection **3**

2 What Happens While You Sleep? **26**

3 The Sleep/Metabolism Matrix **38**

4 The Unique Sleep Challenges of Women **54**

Part II:

Sleep Yourself Thinner: The Plan

5 Diagnose Your Sleep Deficits **81**

6 The 5 Simple Rules for Better Sleep **96**

7 Design the Right Environment **132**

8 Eat Right to Sleep Tight **168**

Part III:

The Sleep Doctor's Diet Plan Recipes 191

Notes 231

Index 241

Foreword

I have a confession to make: I am obsessed with sleep and the dangers of sleep deprivation. A couple of years ago I passed out from exhaustion, broke my cheekbone, and got five stitches over my eye. Ever since then, I've studied the ways sleep affects every aspect of our lives: work, relationships, and, especially, our health. In fact, in 2010 the Huffington Post launched Sleep Challenge in conjunction with *Glamour* magazine, and both editor-in-chief Cindi Leive and I asked our readers to join us in resolving to get more sleep. Michael Breus, the Sleep Doctor, provided medical expertise for the challenge, and his observations on the strong connection between weight loss and sufficient sleep were just one of the many discoveries that came from that challenge—although certainly one that many women will find compelling.

For me, getting enough sleep is much more than a health tip. It helps us access the keys to unlocking the big ideas that will change our world. As I said, my obsession with sleep started with a bang—more like a thud, actually. That was the sound of my face hitting the edge of my desk. It was April 2007. The night before, I arrived home from the airport at midnight, following a week-long tour of colleges with my daughter. I had agreed to her request—okay, it was more like a demand—that there be no checking of my BlackBerry during the day, which meant staying up very late at night catching up on work. That particular morning, I got up just after 5 a.m. to pretape a CNN show. I returned home and, after about an hour, began to feel cold.

Next thing I knew, I was lying on the floor, bloodied. I had passed out from exhaustion and banged my head on the way down. The result was a broken cheekbone and five stitches under my eyebrow.

That's when I knew I needed to mend my estranged relationship with sleep. We had once been quite close, especially early in my career. But, as time went by, responsibilities piled up and we grew apart, taking each other for granted. Sometimes we'd go days and barely see each other. However, when it comes to wakeup calls, few are as effective as the spilling of your own blood.

So sleep is back in my life. And the more I study the issue—and the more I see how sleep deprived we've become as a nation—the more I realize that sleep is, in fact, the next big feminist issue.

Obviously, women have made great strides in all areas of society, especially the workplace. But our national delusion that the way to be ultraproductive is to cut back on sleep is particularly destructive for women. On average, single working women and working mothers actually get 1½ hours less sleep than the minimum 7½ hours the body needs to function.

This, really, is no surprise. Just because women have added responsibilities in the workplace doesn't mean the division of labor at home has changed accordingly.

In the macho boys' club atmosphere that dominates many offices, women too often feel they have to overcompensate by working harder, longer, and later. In fact, lack of sleep has become a sort of virility symbol. I had dinner recently with a guy who kept bragging that he had gotten only 4 hours of sleep the night before. I wanted to tell him—though I didn't—that our dinner would have been a lot more interesting if he had gotten 5. In the cult of no sleep, 7 a.m. is the new 9 a.m. Trying to make a breakfast appointment is now an exercise in sleep deprivation one-upmanship. "Oh, hi, Arianna, yeah, eight is a bit late, but it's fine because that'll give me time to play a few sets of tennis and get in a couple of conference calls to London first."

This has to stop. The scientific research is in—not getting enough sleep is not a sign of virility.

Lack of sleep leads to an increased risk of high blood pressure, obesity, diabetes, weakened immune system, anxiety, depression, and heart disease—the risk for which goes up more for women than for men. Lack of sleep can also, I kid you not, give you a very bad hair day, since the stress of not sleeping accelerates female hair loss. And, as Dr. Breus shows, there is a direct line between the dark circles under your eyes and the extra inches around your waist!

Sleep deprivation is also involved in one of every six fatal car crashes. So, literally, it is killing us. And when it's not killing us, it's turning us into zombies. It's no coincidence, for example, that sleep deprivation is a key strategy of many cults. They force members to stay awake for extended periods because it degrades their decision-making ability and makes them more open to persuasion.

And it's not only decision-making that suffers, but also memory and creativity. Sleep deprivation severely affects relational memory, which is the brain's ability to combine and synthesize distinct facts. It's the sort of thinking that allows us to see the big picture and solve problems with creative and innovative breakthroughs.

But your brain just doesn't do it as well if you don't get enough sleep. Bill Clinton, who famously claimed to survive on only 5 hours of sleep, once admitted, "Every important mistake I've made in my life, I've made because I was too tired."

Do you want more proof? Lack of sleep played a role in the Three Mile Island meltdown, the *Exxon Valdez* oil spill, and the explosion of the *Challenger* space shuttle.

If Lehman Brothers had been Lehman Brothers and Sisters, they might still be around. While the brothers were busy bragging about having gotten only 4 hours of sleep, some Lehman Sister might have noticed the iceberg looming up ahead, because that's the central part of leadership: seeing the icebergs before they hit the *Titanic*.

The prevailing culture tells us nothing succeeds like excess, and that working 70 hours a week is better than working 60. We're told that being plugged in 24/7 is expected, and that sleeping less and multitasking more are an express elevator to the top.

I couldn't disagree more. It's time for us to open our eyes to the value of shutting them.

Arianna Huffington
March 2011

Acknowledgments

I also want to thank the following people.

- My coauthor, Deb Bruce, PhD, without whom this book would never have been written. Thanks for getting this book out of my head and onto the paper.
- Arianna Huffington, for her amazing foreword and for continuing to bring the power of sleep out of the darkness and into the light.
- My father, Alan, who taught me that the key to any accomplishment is persistence. Amen, brother.
- Myra Brown, my business partner, friend, and guardian. Thanks, MB. Without your ideas, coaching, and outlines this book might never have been written.
- The whole Brown family: Dan, Hilary, Phoebe, Lili, and Dr. and Mrs. Goldstein, for putting up with all the crazy hours, stress, and late-night editing your wife, mom, and daughter has had to go through.
- My grandfather, Jack Citronbaum, for living to 101 and still going strong. I think and talk about you all the time.
- Cookie, I think about you all the time, and I miss you very much.
- My agent, Ellen Geiger, at the Frances Goldin Literary Agency, for her neverending, positive attitude and for realizing that so many will benefit from this book.
- My editor, Pam Krauss, who really helped shape my message for all to hear and be able to accomplish their goals.
- Danielle Burch, Sarah Hall, and everyone at Sarah Hall Productions for keeping the faith; I will never forget it.
- Rodale Inc. for all the efforts they have put behind my book and my message.

- Sunny Sea Gold, former *Glamour* health editor, who championed the *Glamour* Sleep Challenge. Thanks for listening.
- Cindi Lieve, editor-in-chief of *Glamour* magazine, for bring the issue of sleep to light for women everywhere.
- All the amazing sleep researchers who contributed to this book, but especially Dr. Eve Van Cauter and Dr. Giovanni Cizza, whose endless search for answers about the sleep-weight relationship was invaluable. Without their tireless work, the field would not be where it is in this important area.
- Pat O'Connor, PhD, and Ileana Arias, PhD. Without you both, I would have never made it through graduate school and learned how to read research and practice psychology.
- Drs. Mehmet Oz and Mike Roizen for your counsel, mentorship, kind words, and friendship. You two are fantastic. Thank you so much for adding to this book.
- My friends at Vemma—BK and Steve—for helping get the word out about this book and for their commitment to better sleep for everyone.
- Drs. Mike Wolff and Dave Berg. Thank you for allowing me to become a better doctor with your patients.
- Everyone at IBC for helping another of my visions come to life. We will change an industry together.
- A special thank you to the Acker family, Neil, and all the Mattress Professionals at Sleepy's.
- All the mattress retailers who share my vision for better sleep.
- Another special thanks to David Perry; I appreciate your honesty, journalism, and friendship. Let's keep changing the game together.
- T-Ham—thanks just for putting up with me! ☺
- Also a big thank-you to Travis Stork, MD; Rosie O'Donnell; and Nan-Kirsten Forte, for your kind words.
- Lastly, Bonnie and Erin. You were right, "That is hot!"

Introduction

As a clinical psychologist who has specialized for the past 14 years in the treatment of sleep disorders, I have seen thousands of patients who arrive at our lab with years of sleep baggage weighing on them and, once they are treated, leave feeling rested and renewed. It has been immensely gratifying to know that I can help people improve their lives and health so quickly and easily simply by improving their sleep.

And while I have treated both men and women during this time, it is often the women who struggle with the most-resistant sleep problems, many of them associated with aging, hormonal imbalances, emotional stress, and sleep hygiene problems. Ironically, these women tend to be healthy in most respects, but they come to me exhausted, sleep deprived, overweight, and unfit. Many of the women have problems associated with obesity, such as hypertension, metabolic syndrome, and type 2 diabetes. Too tired to exercise or be active, they beg for answers that will allow them to sleep well at night so they can feel alert and reclaim their youthful energy.

I'm happy to say that in the great majority of these cases, making changes—often very simple ones—to daily routines and habits as well as the sleep environment has allowed these women to get the quality *and* the quantity of sleep that they have been craving. Without exception these patients have felt better, had an improved outlook on life, felt more energetic, and had fewer "foggy thinking" moments, all of which I had expected to see result from relief of their sleep deprivation. What I had *not* expected to see was that when my female patients slept better, many of them actually lost weight! In some cases, women who came to me with sleep problems caused by being overweight were able to reduce or even eliminate their sleep treatment. To me, this was the ultimate cure!

Take Janet, age 34. The mother of three young boys, she was so sleep deprived that she would snack all day long in an attempt to get more energy. Within a year after giving birth to her youngest son, Janet had gained 15 pounds. This weight gain caused her to snore loudly, prompting her husband to move to the bedroom down the hall.

After running several diagnostic sleep tests, Janet was diagnosed with a mild case of sleep apnea and a big case of insufficient sleep syndrome. Janet started the apnea treatment (CPAP) and used some of the strategies in this book to take control of her sleep quality and sleep quantity. She not only began to feel better, but also showed up for her 3-month follow-up appointment 15 pounds lighter!

Patient stories like Janet's became so common that I started to take a serious look at the critical relationship between poor sleep and being overweight or obese. Further study and a fortuitous meeting at a professional conference led me to researcher Eve Van Cauter, PhD, whose fascinating work in glucose metabolism and sleep deprivation has been critical to my understanding of this complex connection. But that wasn't the end of it. The more I looked into her findings, as well as those of other researchers who were proving the link between *poor* sleep and weight *gain,* the more I began to suspect that *good* sleep and weight *loss* were simply the flip side of the same coin! And this theory was born out time and again in my own practice, with patient after patient shedding unwanted pounds as they improved their sleep patterns.

In late 2009, I was asked to help *Glamour* magazine conduct a sleep challenge for their readers using the elements of the sleep program I recommend for my clients. When I mentioned to the writer offhandedly that I could almost guarantee their readers would lose weight if they followed my program, her reaction was telling: She stopped scribbling notes, looked me directly in the eyes, and exclaimed, "Really!"

I tried to explain the complicated sleep research, but all she was interested in was the distinct possibility of losing weight by sleeping more. The editor at *Glamour* asked if we could put some women through a test—using a simple set of sleep rules—to see if they felt better and had more energy after getting better sleep.

When the results of the *Glamour* Sleep Challenge hit the newsstands in March of 2009, the response was huge. Not only had seven out of eight women lost between 3 and 15 pounds, but newer and more comprehensive research that had been recently published had also helped me devise other strategies to augment the sleep–weight-loss effect. As my patients used these different sleep strategies, the pounds seemed almost to melt off—even when the patients didn't adopt a restrictive weight-loss diet or amp up their fitness regimens!

With all this information in mind, I realized that I had a powerful message to bring to women everywhere—that good sleep is not only important for their mental and physical health, but also necessary to help them lose weight or maintain a healthy weight. Of course, different women will have different results, but I can assure you of one thing: *If you follow the Sleep Doctor's 5 Simple Rules, your sleep, weight, and health will improve.* The guidelines I outline in the pages that follow can be used in conjunction with any diet plan you may currently be following, and they work in any situation.

In Part I, I will give you a greater understanding of how sleep is related to your weight, your health, and your looks and how obstacles such as chronic stress and changing female hormones can disrupt a good night's sleep. Then, you can set yourself up for a great night's sleep in Part II. Using the Sleep Diary explained in Chapters 4 and 5, you will identify the stumbling blocks that prevent you from getting good sleep.

Then, in Chapters 6 through 8, you will learn the *Sleep Doctor's 5 Simple Rules* (page 96) and practical strategies to help you take control of both your sleep and your weight. In Part III, I will provide you with some scrumptious recipes that are filled with nutritional compounds that boost calmness and relaxation, making it easier to fall asleep and stay asleep.

My goal is to help you find the right tools to sleep soundly every night and, in doing so, to drop unwanted pounds and find your ideal weight. Based on the latest scientific research and my patients' experiences, I am convinced that better sleep will allow you to feel more emotionally balanced, boost your self-esteem, and help you look great as the extra pounds come off. Moreover, unlike virtually every other weight-loss program out there, mine requires *no deprivation whatsoever.* In fact, many people would consider the only requirement for this plan an indulgence: Get more and better sleep! All I'm asking you to sacrifice are the dark circles under your eyes and the gnawing sense of fatigue you have been dragging around with you, perhaps for years.

Sound too good to be true? Read on. You'll soon discover, as I did, that there have never been more compelling reasons to put sleep first. So fluff up your pillow, adjust your reading light, and let's start knocking down those obstacles between you and a great night's sleep—and your favorite skinny jeans—right now.

Part I

The Science of
SLEEP
Meets the Science of
WEIGHT LOSS

1

The Sleep/Weight
Connection

If you're like most women with a few pounds to lose, you've probably tried just about everything to rid yourself of that unwanted weight. Perhaps you've experimented with a low-carb or low-fat diet or an eating plan that severely restricts calories, or maybe you've amped up your fitness routine, and yet those unwanted pounds hang on stubbornly. But there's one thing I bet you haven't tried in your battle of the bulge, and that is getting more sleep.

Think about it. How incredible would it be if the only change you had to make to your routine in order to drop 5, 10, or even more pounds was to get an extra hour of sleep? No more cabbage soup. No high-fiber wafers or extra Spin classes—just 1 more hour of restorative, restful sleep each and every day. Who in the world (including your doctor, by the way) would object to that?

But can sleep possibly be an effective diet aid? Can something so benign, so sustainable—so inexpensive!—with absolutely no unwanted side effects possibly get you the results that all the deprivation diets and long hours at the gym have failed to achieve? The research is clear and conclusive: Giving your body the rest it needs will enable you to lose weight *even if you do not alter your diet or fitness routine.* Furthermore, no matter how conscientious you are about what you eat and how active you are, a poor sleep pattern is likely to torpedo your good intentions and allow those extra pounds to creep onto your body and stay there!

I wrote *The Sleep Doctor's Diet Plan* to help you understand your unique relationship with sleep and what good sleep can do to improve your weight, your health, and how you feel about yourself. I want you to learn ways to regain control in your nightly sleep battle or to simply make your good sleep even better so you can either achieve the healthy weight you want or prevent the gradual accumulation of fat around the waist that so inevitably seems to occur as we age.

Sleep Is the Missing Link

In my clinical practice, I treat hundreds of women who come to me with complaints of poor sleep and an inability to lose weight. Most women tell of having either difficulty sleeping (whether it's falling asleep or staying asleep) or poor-quality sleep.

My sleep patients also say, "You don't understand what I am going through, trying to lose weight. Nothing works," but I really do understand. As a clinical psychologist who is board certified in clinical sleep disorders, I have treated many women who have the same problem—an inability to sleep combined with *an inability to make the scale budge,* despite trying every diet—low carb, low fat, and low calorie.

The reality is that women face different situations in life that cause their weight gain—ranging from ongoing family or career stress to ignoring the importance of daily exercise to hormonal changes at midlife that pack on the pounds—and most will have a hard time reversing that weight gain. This can be frustrating, especially when you try to stick with a popular diet and exercise regimen that's "guaranteed" to bring success.

But I have discovered that there is a "missing link" in most trendy weight-loss diets and it has *nothing* to do with what you eat or how many miles you log on your treadmill each day. In fact, this missing link provides women of all ages with a tool for dealing with what the surgeon general calls "America's obesity crisis." ***That missing link is proper and adequate sleep.***

After sorting through the ever-mounting stacks of scientific literature, I have identified a clear-cut connection between poor sleep and obesity. In a nutshell, both insufficient sleep and poor-quality sleep make your body want to store fat, not burn it! Moreover, I have discovered that the best way to decrease your weight is to increase good-quality sleep in conjunction with following a balanced weight-loss diet. And even without changing the food you eat or exercising vigorously, simply getting better sleep can help you lose weight or maintain a normal weight. In this book, I will teach you how to boost your metabolic rate, decrease your appetite, and lose weight simply by improving your sleep quality and quantity.

Here's why. During deep sleep, your brain secretes a large amount of growth hormone, which tells your body how to break down fat for fuel. If you don't allow your body to get enough deep sleep, there won't be enough growth hormone to break down the fat that results when you take in extra calories. Instead, your body takes a shortcut and packs the added fat away in your thighs, belly, or butt—wherever you tend to gain weight. In addition, poor sleep appears to increase your appetite. And what an appetite you will have: You'll crave sweets, carbs, and high-fat foods.

As a researcher and a practicing sleep doctor, I use both scientific data and information from my patients to help me develop therapies for the people who seek treatment at my sleep clinic. No matter how many diets my patients have tried (and failed at) in the past, I find that they won't lose the extra weight and keep it off until they ***relearn how to get better sleep.***

I know what you're thinking: Between kids, career, and commitments, who really has time for more sleep? For most women, there's always one more thing to do—one more lunch to make, one more client to e-mail, one more problem to worry about. All too often, sleep becomes the last priority on your to-do list. But if sleep becomes a hit-or-miss proposition for you, it's more than likely that the eventual result will be a gradual—potentially permanent—weight gain.

There is no doubt that consistently getting a good night's sleep is a familiar battle in our society today. Perhaps you know from experience how a lack of sleep can wreak havoc on your energy level and performance. The problem arises when you get inadequate sleep day after day. You will not only experience a lack of energy and an inability to focus during the day, but also start to notice that your waistband is snugger, your jeans feel tighter, and the number on the bathroom scale is inching higher. *Believe me when I say that these occurrences are no coincidence!* Recent research has found that people who sleep less have a *slower metabolic rate* (the speed at which your body burns calories and the rate that we all want to raise!). Metabolism is the body's process for turning calories into energy, and it varies at different sleep stages. For instance, REM is the sleep stage during which metabolism is the highest. *If you get less sleep, you get less REM sleep, too.* This sets the stage for eating the wrong foods, eating too much food, and eating at the wrong time of day (or night).

Good Sleep Is Essential— Every Night

You know that even occasional sleep problems make a normal day more stressful and less productive. That's because your body and mind need consistent, restful sleep to function optimally. Remember, sleep is not a luxury or a treat, like splurging on dessert. *Sleep is a necessary physiological function that keeps you alive.* Let's take a look at how missing just *1 night* of shut-eye affects your looks, your mind, and your health.

- Your skin looks pasty, your eyes get puffy, and poor hydration makes your under-eye circles more pronounced.

- Your prefrontal cortex shuts down. This is the part of your brain that controls logical reasoning and the "fight-or-flight" response. You instantly become a poor decision maker. As a result, your choices of foods lean toward comfort foods (i.e., high carbs and high fat) to increase your level of serotonin (the calming hormone), and you're apt to skip the gym because of fatigue.

- Your insulin production increases and your body starts to store fat more easily. Over time, this can lead to serious illnesses such as obesity, hypertension, and type 2 diabetes.

- You have problems completing tasks, whether simple or complex.

- Your ability to speak and remember diminishes as your brain is depleted of its ability to consolidate memories.

- You become irritable, possibly even irrational.

- You have difficulty focusing and concentrating.

- Your muscles ache, making movement difficult.

Chances are, you recognize most of these symptoms. But now imagine weeks to months of poor sleep and how this can lead to premature aging, weight gain, and even a larger abdomen. I see the following problems almost daily in my female patients.

Poor Complexion and Bad Hair

Poor sleep can make you look older. You can see the effects of sleep loss when you look in your bathroom mirror in the morning. Lack of sleep can make your skin look swollen and ashen and can accentuate the deep reddish blue color under your eyes (dark circles). In addition, because sleep deprivation leads to poor circulation (circulation is how hair and skin get their nutrients), poor sleep is linked to facial wrinkles and thinning hair.

PROBLEMS LINKED TO SLEEP LOSS

PROBLEM AREA	WHAT YOU MIGHT NOTICE	WHAT YOU MIGHT NOT NOTICE
WEIGHT GAIN AND EVENTUAL OBESITY	• Increased hunger • Weight gain	• A lower level of the "stop eating" hormone, leptin • A higher level of the "go get some food" hormone, ghrelin • A lower level of serotonin, a calming neurotransmitter
BAD SKIN AND HAIR	• Puffy, pasty skin • Thinning skin • Facial wrinkles • Reddish blue under-eye circles • Thinning hair • Complete hair loss	• Skin dehydration • Skin that's more susceptible to bacteria and allergens • Premature aging
PAIN	• Increased pain sensitivity • Sore muscles • Joint pain	• A lower level of serotonin, which can increase pain • Increased blood levels of pro-inflammatory markers, which are signs of systemic inflammation • Increased pain that is caused by inflammation
FOCUS AND MEMORY	• Low energy • Inability to focus • Impulsivity	• Changes in mental functioning • Imbalanced neurotransmitter levels
TYPE 2 DIABETES	• Elevated blood sugar • Frequent urination • Eye and skin infections	• Hypertension • Increased risk of heart attack • Damage to kidneys, eyes, and other organs

In a study reported in the *Journal of Investigative Dermatology,* researchers tested sleep-deprived women and found that their skin was more susceptible to outside allergens and bacteria.[1] For some women, lack of sleep can worsen acne, rosacea, and dermatitis. Other studies have shown that poor sleep ultimately reduces immunity and results in skin that is dehydrated, wrinkled, pale, and unable to repair itself quickly. In a recent study, scientists in Sweden found that sleep deprived people look less healthy, more tired, and less attractive than people who get a full night's sleep.[2]

PROBLEM AREA	WHAT YOU MIGHT NOTICE	WHAT YOU MIGHT NOT NOTICE
HIGH BLOOD PRESSURE AND HEART DISEASE	• Increased blood pressure • Insomnia • Waking up with shortness of breath • Daytime fatigue • Signs of heart disease • Heart failure	• Sleep apnea and periodic breathing • Type 2 diabetes
MOODINESS AND DEPRESSION	• Irritability • Lethargy • High anxiety • Decreased sex drive • Depression • Memory loss • Negligence • Reduced performance	• Less REM sleep • A lower level of serotonin in the brain • Altered levels of neurotransmitters that regulate mood
IMMUNE DYSFUNCTION	• Increased viral and bacterial infections	• Inflammatory arthritis or asthma • An increased risk for cancer

Pain in the Neck, Back, and . . . You Name It!

A National Sleep Foundation *Sleep in America* poll found that one in four women has pain or physical discomfort that interrupts her sleep three nights a week or more.[3] Did you know that poor sleep causes greater pain sensitivity? Sleeplessness leads to a lower level of the neurotransmitter serotonin in the body, and these lower levels can increase pain perception. An increase in the serotonin level in the brain is associated with a calming, anxiety-reducing effect, and in some cases drowsiness. When serotonin is depleted from lack of sleep, the result is an increase in pain sensitivity, as well as increased feelings of anxiety, malaise, and even depression.

So how does your body increase its serotonin production? By telling you to eat foods that are high in carbohydrates, an effect that is often magnified by your having a high level of the stress hormone cortisol, which also increases your appetite for carbs. This is a vicious cycle!

Moodiness and Depression

Poor sleep can cause you to have mood swings and increased anxiety, and it can even lead to depression in some women. Between 65 and 75 percent of the patients I see in clinics have either anxiety or depression as both a cause and a result of their sleep problems. It's not uncommon for patients with sleep deprivation to report bad moods, irritability, fatigue, decreased sex drive, and other signs of psychological dysfunction. The good news is that many of these symptoms usually lessen in severity or even disappear when good sleep habits are reestablished.

Focus and Memory Problems

Daytime sleepiness results in lower concentration, poor short-term memory, and decreased productivity. Your energy level and attention to detail are both compromised by poor sleep. Some women who experience frequent sleep deprivation wonder if they have attention deficit/hyperactivity disorder (ADHD), a problem that is associated with an inability to focus or pay attention and sometimes with impulsivity. But most of these women do not have ADHD; they are simply too sleepy to focus and pay attention.

Reduced Immunity (Getting Sicker Quicker)

Sleep plays a big role in regulating your immune system, and a weakened immune system can result in ailments such as viral and bacterial infections. From scientific studies, we know that exposure to viruses and bacteria results in no health problems—*if* your immune system is strong. Yet when faced with sleep deprivation, the immune system cannot work at full capacity.[4] When your immune system malfunctions, you are at risk for autoimmune diseases such as inflammatory arthritis, allergies, and asthma. When the immune system is weak, bacteria, viruses, and toxicity can overwhelm the body.

Less Sleep = Weight Gain

You now know that along with having a direct correlation with obesity, poor sleep also has very serious physical and mental health consequences. So, here's a simple question: *How much sleep do you average each night?* Do you get more than 8 hours a night, or are you lucky to squeeze in 6 to 7 hours of sleep? Chronic sleep deprivation is very common in the United States today. In fact, even though sleep doctors recommend 7 to 9 hours of sleep per night, adults in the United States average only 6.85 hours per night, and *30 percent of adults get less than 6 hours of sleep each night*.[5, 6]

At the same time, the prevalence of obesity (having a body mass index, or BMI, of 30 or higher) in the United States has rapidly increased over the past 3 decades. Scientists are now convinced that increased sleep deprivation is related to the obesity epidemic.[7, 8] See the chart below and I think you will see an interesting trend.

Increase in Obesity Parallels Decrease in Sleep Time

	OBESITY RATE IN U.S. ADULTS[9]	AVERAGE SLEEP TIME IN U.S. ADULTS
1960	13.4%	8–8.9 hours[10]
1995	23.2%	7 hours[11]
2005*	32.7%	6.9 hours[12]
2010	35%+	6.5 hours

In 2005, the National Center for Health Statistics reported that 30 percent of adults were getting less than 6 hours of sleep per night.

The *decrease* in average sleep duration in the United States has occurred over the same time period as the *increases* in the prevalence of obesity; metabolic syndrome (a constellation of conditions that increase the chances of developing cardiovascular disease and type 2 diabetes); and type 2 diabetes, a disease in which blood glucose levels are abnormally high.[13, 14] While the latest sleep research cannot prove this conclusively, there appears to be a relationship.

Good Sleep, Bad Sleep, No Sleep

Still, you may think it's quite *normal* to sleep no longer than 6 or 7 hours. After all, most of your friends get little sleep, so why not? In reality, up until the 19th century, it was *normal* for women and men alike to sleep as much as 10 hours each night. Then gas lamps were invented in the 1790s and, in the 1880s, Thomas Edison perfected the lightbulb. Since Edison's bright invention, the number of hours Americans sleep has declined sharply.

Another development that dramatically affected sleep habits in America was the introduction of overtime. When people learned that they could earn more money by working more hours, they started to let sleep slide.[15] Since then, American workers have been clocking more and more hours on the job and now work more hours than individuals in most other industrialized nations do.[16] More income may sound good, but the problem with constantly working more than 40 hours a week is what overworking does to your mind and body. Fatigue, stress, and health problems such as hypertension, heart disease, and obesity become common. Spending more hours at work results in less time with the family, less time for pleasure . . . and *less time for sleep.*

Anxiety Robs You of Good Sleep

Anxiety is a major sleep robber, especially for women. Between 65 and 75 percent of the patients I see in clinics have either anxiety or depression, which fuels their sleep problems. In short, they can't turn their active minds off. Even if they do doze off eventually, they say they sleep restlessly most of the night, worrying and ruminating about their lives.

Anxiety is a normal feeling that helps motivate us to act in certain situations that require heightened awareness of our thoughts or behaviors.[17] For example, imagine that you are driving to work and suddenly the car in front of you stops without warning. Adrenaline floods your body and causes your reaction time to speed up, helping you to quickly slam on the brakes. Another example of beneficial anxiety is when you have a tight deadline at work. It's very common to feel a great sense of anxiety or worry until the project is completed, at which point you can breathe deeply and relax again.

For some women, anxiety gets out of control. The anxiety comes and goes without warning, and seemingly without reason. Some women have anxiety so severe that they experience panic attacks, during which their hearts race and their throats feel like they're closing in so they cannot breathe. Panic attacks are extremely debilitating, but they are highly treatable, so ask your doctor for help if you experience them.

Sometimes anxiety is more subtle. Worry is a form of anxiety that seems to affect many of my sleep patients. Worry can come in many forms, from flat-out panic to a subtle feeling of nervousness experienced as you go over your to-do list for the next day.

There are several different anxiety disorders, including phobias, social anxiety, and other types, that can be diagnosed and treated by medical and mental health professionals. It is important to know that these anxiety conditions, though distressing, can be treated and controlled with medication and/or behavioral interventions.[18] If you believe that your anxiety is out of control or negatively affecting your sleep, make an appointment to discuss this with your medical doctor.[19]

BORN TO WORRY?

A 2005 Gallup poll showed a significant difference between the number of women and the number of men who claimed to be worried "a great deal" about current issues.[20] Researchers believe that part of this is due to how women are wired: Women's brains process information and emotions differently than men's brains do. Fortunately, neuroscience is making huge strides in understanding how and why these brain differences occur, but for now scientists are aware that sex differences between brains do exist.

Many believe that women are different from men biologically. Others hypothesize that women and men are socialized to interpret and cope with stressors differently. Some say that women are better multitaskers than men are. Perhaps because women are so good at multitasking, they tend to take on more responsibilities than their male counterparts do.

However, because a woman's body produces stress hormones differently, women can become more taxed over time than men do. That's when women start to ruminate, or repeatedly mull over problems. It's not uncommon for women to play scenarios over and over in their minds. Sure, the problems remain unresolved, but the images keep repeating themselves.

If you have problems with rumination at bedtime, allow yourself a full 5 minutes during the daytime hours to obsess about and explore the scenario that is causing you worry and anxiety. When the timer goes off, stop. Change rooms, drink some tea, and do something to take your mind off the problem. Don't get caught up in the rumination cycle, because this is a surefire sleep destroyer.

Internet Addiction Disturbs Sleep

The most recent sleep robber that has impacted millions so dramatically is the Internet. Spending hour after hour searching for cool stuff on eBay or checking out old high school friends on Facebook moves your brain further away from sleep. As you gaze at the computer screen, your brain awakens, the electrical activity increases, and the neurons start to race.[21, 22] This is the *exact opposite* of what should be happening in your brain before bedtime.

In addition, we think the blue light on your computer monitor (not to mention that on some of the new handheld devices) can have a negative effect on your biological circadian rhythm. Even small amounts of light from a monitor (or a cell phone) can pass through the retina of the eye into part of the hypothalamus (the part of the brain that controls sleep activities) and delay the pineal gland's release of melatonin,[23] the hormone that is necessary for sleep.

On a side note, sunlight is an exceptional source of blue light. Sunlight is a blend of different colors, including blue light. This explains why you feel more alert when you go outside on a sunny day. You need sunlight and specifically blue light during the daytime hours—but not in the evening—in order to produce melatonin and feel sleepy at night.

Secretion of melatonin by the pineal gland peaks in the middle of the night and then gradually falls, reaching its lowest level by morning.

Feeling Tired Is Not Normal

Even after lengthy discussions about the need to resolve sleep disruptions such as nighttime worrying and Internet addiction, many of my patients simply will not accept that *being tired is not normal.* They complain of having *no time to sleep,* explaining that they spend so much time working, commuting, and parenting that they simply cannot squeeze in 1 more minute to relax and sleep each night. Researchers confirm this, concluding that our work-driven culture keeps us from getting the rest we need.[24] And even when we read studies showing that more sleep will reenergize our bodies and minds and help us maintain a normal weight, it's still hard to stop burning the candle at both ends. My patients tell of having the following sleep problems.

- Waking up every night at 3:00 a.m., then feeling exhausted the following day
- Not being able to turn off their minds when they get into bed
- Having a snoring bed partner who keeps them up all night and irritable
- Waking up frequently throughout the night

Take my patient Lana, 37, for example. She came to see me for help with her inability to fall asleep easily and stay asleep. As much as she tried to relax, Lana would lie awake for hours, ruminating over everything she had failed to do that day. In addition, she was frustrated by her failure to lose a single pound after following a strict low-carb diet for 6 weeks. When I asked her about other lifestyle factors that might be causing her sleep problems, she admitted that she was overly stressed about her job and found no time to exercise during the day or to relax during the evening hours. After assessing Lana's discussion, it became apparent to me that her unhealthy lifestyle habits, including too much stress and too little exercise, were keeping her from getting enough good-quality sleep, which was stalling her weight loss.

Lana was shocked to learn that her inability to sleep for longer than 6 hours a night was affecting her weight, since she was fairly compliant with a carb-restricted diet. I explained to her that sleep does not have an on/off switch and that she had to follow some basic rules to get her body ready for nighttime slumber. I gave Lana the necessary tools to get better sleep, and the pounds started rolling off.

Tamara's Night Sweats Kept Her on High Alert

I have treated hundreds of women who sleep restlessly during the natural transitions of perimenopause and menopause. These women not only complain of night sweats and hot flashes, but most also want to know how to lose the extra 10 pounds that often accompany menopause.

What if your problem is not too little sleep, but rather sleeping too much? Here we have a sleep-quality problem. This means that there is something affecting the quality of your sleep. My patient Rosa is a perfect example.

Rosa came to see me because her husband was complaining about her snoring. She was shy about admitting it because she felt it was not very feminine, but she could snore with the best of them. As it turned out, Rosa had also had a weight problem for most of her adult life. After a clinical evaluation and a formal sleep study, Rosa was diagnosed with sleep apnea, a sleep disorder that causes you to unknowingly stop breathing hundreds of times each night and awakens you momentarily each time in order to breathe again. She was placed on a CPAP—continuous positive airway pressure—machine to help her breathe throughout the night. The CPAP machine blew air into her collapsed throat, helping to keep it open so she could breathe and stay asleep. Once she adjusted to the sleep apnea treatment (and it did take about 4 to 5 weeks), she began to see her sleep improve. In fact, she reported to me that she had more energy and—oddly enough, she thought—was less hungry. When I saw Rosa at her 6-month follow-up appointment, she had lost 25 pounds through diet and better sleep and I was able to adjust her treatment.

Tamara, 52, came to see me about sleep and weight problems. She had high anxiety about going to bed at night because of hormone-related night sweats that left her hot, damp, and then freezing cold. I gave Tamara information on moisture-wicking, breathable pajamas to prevent the moisture from night sweats from staying on her skin and making her cold. Also, I encouraged her to increase the temperature in her room, so that when she did sweat, the moisture would not make her as cold, which had been causing her to awaken. Tamara tried these sleep solutions, and within a few days she was sleeping a little more than 7.5 hours a night with minimal disturbances. At her next visit 2 months later, Tamara said *she'd lost 8 pounds* without making any intentional changes in her diet, although she said she had stopped snacking between meals because she was no longer feeling weak and hungry. Once again: *Better sleep = weight loss!*

It's remarkable to hear the reactions of patients like Tamara after they improve their sleep and, as a consequence, also experience weight loss. While we don't have all the answers about the link between sleep and weight and why women have very specific concerns, we do know that women who are in tune with their bodies' need for sleep can maintain a normal, healthy weight and optimal wellness.

The Dangers of Sleep Deprivation

As a clinician who has studied the ramifications of sleep loss and disruption for more than a decade and conducted numerous sleep studies, I have seen very clearly that simple fatigue is merely the tip of the iceberg. And I'm far from alone in making these observations; fascinating new studies are being published each month supporting the theory that lack of sleep leads to obesity and related problems such as metabolic syndrome, diabetes, hypertension, and other health conditions. Here are some of the most interesting recent findings.

Lack of Sleep Makes You Fatter

In the Nurses' Health Study, 70,026 women were studied to see whether not sleeping enough increased the risk of future weight gain and even obesity. Researchers concluded that self-reported sleep restriction impacts your ability to burn calories and increases the risk of weight gain. In fact, they reported that women in the study who slept 7 to 8 hours per night had the lowest risk for major weight gain. Similar studies suggest that those who sleep less than 7 hours per night are more likely to be obese.[25]

In a study of middle-aged women, researchers concluded that weight gain was directly correlated with the amount of sleep the subjects received each night. This study started about 20 years ago and included more than 68,000 women who were asked every 2 years about their sleep patterns as well as their weight. After 16 years, the findings revealed that those women who slept 5 hours or less each night weighed 5.4 pounds more than the women who slept 7 hours. In addition, women who slept 5 or fewer hours per night were 15 percent more likely to become obese than women who slept 7 hours each night.[26] Another sleep study reported that losing just 16 minutes of sleep per night increased the risk of obesity.[27]

Lack of Sleep Makes You Eat More Carbs and Snacks

In a revealing study, scientists at the University of Chicago allowed people to sleep 5.5 hours on 1 night and 8.5 on another and then measured how many free snacks they downed the next day.[28] The participants ate an average of 221 calories *more* when sleepy—an amount that could translate into almost a pound gained in 2 weeks!

In another study that reviewed short sleep (less than 6 hours) in young adults, researchers concluded that after poor sleep, the increase in appetite for foods with high carbohydrate content was particularly strong. It was as if the sleep-deprived brain craved its primary fuel, glucose, which your body produces from carbs.[29]

In addition, not getting enough sleep affects the amounts and types of food you eat. Some studies show that sleeping for a shorter time and spending waking hours in an environment where people tend to overeat can cause you to engage in excessive snacking—and I don't mean on fresh fruits and vegetables.[30]

Lack of Sleep Increases Inflammation and the Risk of Diabetes

Sleeping too little for just one night can increase proinflammatory markers in the blood and boost hunger-promoting chemicals. Studies show that inflammation provoked by certain immune cells leads to insulin resistance and type 2 diabetes. Type 2 diabetes is directly correlated to obesity and is epidemic worldwide. There is increasing evidence that people who sleep fewer than 7 hours a night have a higher risk of diabetes. Researchers at the University of Chicago found that losing just 3 to 4 hours of sleep over a period of several days is enough to trigger metabolic changes that are consistent with a prediabetic state. They determined that when sleep was restricted to 4 hours for 6 consecutive nights, the body's ability to keep blood glucose at a consistent level declined significantly,[31] which increases the risk of type 2 diabetes. This may be because sleep deprivation stresses the body. Getting good-quality sleep is now considered a basic defense mechanism for staying healthy and preventing obesity and type 2 diabetes.[32]

Lack of Sleep Leads to High Blood Pressure

Studies report a link between high blood pressure and sleep deprivation. When people are sleep deprived, whether it is from insufficient sleep *quantity* or poor sleep *quality,* they place an increased load on their hearts.[33] Here's why: When you are awake, your heart pumps faster to move the blood around. During sleep, your body does not require that much bloodflow, so your heart rate slows and the heart gets a much-needed rest. Without ample resting time, the heart muscle gets fatigued. Because your heart has to work harder, you can have an increase in blood pressure or possibly thickening of the heart muscle, which can lead to more serious heart problems.

Lack of Sleep Leads to Metabolic Disturbances

In a study of shift workers with irregular sleep, researchers found that the volunteers had definite *metabolic disturbances* that are clearly linked to insulin resistance. Insulin, a hormone released by the pancreas, promotes the storage of calories as fat and regulates the glucose level in the blood. Metabolic syndrome—also called insulin resistance syndrome—happens when your body steadily becomes less responsive to the actions of insulin. With metabolic syndrome, your blood sugar level rises despite the blood's high level of insulin, and type 2 diabetes can result.[34, 35, 36]

Start Now: Change Your Sleep and Your Weight

Maybe you think you're exhausted, irritable, and overweight because your kids wear you down, causing you to "stress eat" all day long. Or you may think reduced energy and a bigger waistline are just part of growing older. Quite honestly, some women tell me they've *always had sleep and weight problems,* so these issues may go undiagnosed and untreated for years—or even a lifetime.

Starting now, your sleep can be changed. Reading this book is your *first step* toward finally losing weight by making the necessary changes to get better sleep.

Moreover, some groundbreaking reports are suggesting that another aspect of resolving sleep issues can also play a part in weight loss: *Sleep more and you'll eat less—and weigh less.* This is true for a number of reasons. First, in a society with readily available foods and beverages, the longer we are awake, the more likely we are to eat and/or drink. *Sleeping more will likely reduce your calorie intake, especially if you are a nighttime snacker.*

One revealing study reports that by replacing 1 waking hour (say, of watching TV) with an equivalent amount of sleep, we forgo consumption of a significant amount of food because of the resulting reduction in the opportunity to eat. Some reports theorize that eliminating just 125 calories a day (by sleeping *instead of snacking*) can result in a weight loss of 10 pounds over 1 year—with no other dietary modifications of any kind.[37]

The *Glamour* Sleep Challenge

Recently, to test my sleep diet hypothesis, another doctor and I worked with *Glamour* magazine and recruited women to help us investigate the link between sleep and weight loss. In the *Glamour* Sleep Challenge, we gave the participants some simple instructions.

- Get 7.5 hours of sleep on the same schedule each night.
- Start a bedtime routine.
- Reduce your caffeine and alcohol intake if they are high.
- Experiment with exactly how much sleep you need.
- Continue with your normal eating habits and exercise routine.

The women agreed to follow these strategies and to ensure that they were sleeping at least *7.5 hours* each night. That's it. We didn't ask them to make any changes to their eating habits or exercise routines. And the results were clear: *Longer sleep allowed them to lose weight.*

The participants in the *Glamour* magazine sleep challenge ranged in age from 25 to 35. After 8 weeks, six of our participants had lost an average of almost 10 pounds (between 3 and 15 pounds). At the 2-month mark, one woman said her belly was flatter and her love handles were smaller. But get this! At the end of 10 weeks, this same participant had lost almost 5 inches from her waist, hips, bust, and thighs—even though she was not considered overweight to start with. Another volunteer was unable to stick to the sleep diet due to her hectic schedule and did not lose any weight. Still, she lost inches off her bust, waist, and hips. These women not only lost weight, but also actually *felt* better! Their moods were generally better—they did not snap at their family or friends—and they reported feeling healthier.

The *Glamour* Sleep Challenge may also have resulted in weight loss by curbing fatigue-induced cravings. In addition, it may have helped to balance the women's hormones (specifically the hunger-regulating hormones ghrelin and leptin), thus helping them tame their appetites.

The *Glamour* Sleep Challenge participants boasted of the positive changes they observed: Their clothes fit better, they were proud of their leaner figures, and they had increased energy and improved self-esteem. Some of the women had so much more energy that they voluntarily increased their workouts, without our even asking them to! This sleep challenge helped me to develop the key elements of *The Sleep Doctor's Diet Plan,* and started my search for the most important rules for quality sleep.

Calories In versus Calories Out

So why did we see such tremendous results with the *Glamour* study? You probably understand the basic truth of dieting—that you lose weight when the number of calories you consume is less than the number of calories you burn. But why doesn't this equation always work? Why do many women diet every day of their lives and **never lose a pound**?

The reason is that losing weight is not simply a matter of calories in–calories out. The latest studies confirm that weight loss is a far more complex physiological process that is highly influenced by sleep. Once you understand the relationship between your sleep and your weight, you can maximize weight loss by combining the strategies in *The Sleep Doctor's Diet Plan* with those of any diet plan—be it a low-calorie, low-carb, low-glycemic, or low-fat diet, or indeed, no diet at all! In addition, when you add more sleep time, you will receive other benefits, such as increased energy, greater productivity, and a boost in your growth hormone production (not to mention an increase in self-esteem from the weight loss).

Unlike other weight-loss "boosters," adding 30 minutes to 1 hour to your nightly sleep regimen will have absolutely no negative side effects. In fact, the most common side effects of sleeping a little longer are overwhelmingly desirable and positive: increased energy, alertness, and productivity and better relationships at home and at work.

Can *The Sleep Doctor's Diet Plan* Help You?

By now you are wondering if *The Sleep Doctor's Diet Plan* can help you lose weight and feel good about yourself again. There is only one sure way to find out: After you learn more about sleep in Chapter 2, move on to Chapter 3 and learn about the intricate links between sleep, hormones, and your weight. Then read in Chapter 4 about the special problems women have in getting great sleep. You'll then be ready to move on to Part II—and to begin to implement the easy-to-use tools I describe. Following easy strategies, you can:

- Stop the excessive food cravings that are making you lose control of your eating habits and weight
- Gain more control over daytime (and nighttime) snacking
- Learn how to calm down and turn off the fight-or-flight stress response that keeps you wide awake at night

!SLEEP !ALERT

Studies on children reveal the same pattern of chronic sleep restriction and increased weight gain that we are seeing in adults, leaving them at risk for being overweight or even obese at an early age. Experts believe that parents should be educated about the importance of sleep to their kids' health and the harmful effects of sleep loss on children's weight and long-term health. The best thing parents can do? Model healthy sleep behaviors themselves.[38] If kids are going to get adequate sleep each night, moms and dads need to turn the lights off and go to bed early, too.

How much sleep do children need?

Infants

Up to 3 months: 15 hours (10 at night and 5 during the day in three naps)

3 to 6 months: 14.5 hours (11 at night and 3.5 during the day in two naps)

6 to 9 months: 14 hours (11 at night and 3 during the day in two naps)

Toddlers

9 to 12 months: 13.75 hours (11 hours at night and 2.75 hours during the day in two naps)

1 to 1.5 years: 13.5 hours (11.5 hours at night and 2 hours during the day in one nap)

1.5 to 2 years: 13 hours (11 hours at night and 2 hours during the day in one nap)

Preschoolers

2 to 3 years: 12 hours (11 hours at night and 1 hour during the day in one nap)

3 to 5 years: 11.5 hours at night—no daytime sleep or napping

- Become the master of your sleep as you create a personal sleep sanctuary in your bedroom

Hard to believe these simply improve the qualty and duration of your sleep each night? Read on.

Elementary school-age children

5 to 8 years: 11 to 10.5 hours
8 to 11 years: 10.25 to 9.75 hours
11 to 14 years: 9.5 to 9.25 hours

Teens

14 to 16 years: 8.5 to 9 hours
16+ years: 8.5 hours[39]

New studies report that teenagers who get less than 8 hours of sleep each night are more likely to eat high-fat diets. We know that diets high in fat increase the risks for obesity, diabetes, heart disease, and some cancers. A study published in the journal *Sleep* reported that when teenagers are sleep deprived, they eat 2.2 percent more snack and fat calories than teens who sleep 8 or more hours each night do.[40] Accordinging to the National Sleep Foundation, the average teen needs 9.25 hours of sleep each night, but only about 15 percent of teenagers get even 8.5 hours of sleep.[41]

In the *Sleep* study, teens who slept **less than 8 hours a night ate about 1,968 calories** per day. Teens who slept **8 hours or more ate about 250 calories less** (about 1,723 calories a day). The findings of this study are the tip of the iceberg when it comes to understanding why our nation's teens are so overweight. Researchers believe that teenagers' lack of sleep affects their metabolism by changing their levels of leptin and ghrelin, the hormones that control appetite. Teens who get little sleep also have more time to eat high-fat snacks, which adds more calories to their day.

To help them feel alert and rested, make sure your teenagers get at least 9 hours of sleep each night.

2

What Happens While
You Sleep?

To understand why getting enough good-quality sleep is so important to maintaining a healthy weight—not to mention a host of other health considerations—it's useful to know a little bit about sleep itself. Have you ever wondered what really happens when you sleep? After all, you can't watch yourself sleep. Even if you could, you wouldn't be able to see the well-orchestrated physiological processes that occur during sleep without some fairly sophisticated equipment. Before I explain how sleep loss could possibly be to blame for your weight gain or dieting failure, let's start with two simple questions about sleep that have somewhat complex answers.

1. What is sleep supposed to look like?
2. What happens when you sleep?

Even though sleep seems like a passive process, it's not. Sleep is an *active state* that is as complex as wakefulness. Your brain doesn't shut down during sleep; rather, your brain is involved in a wide variety of activities.

The Stages of Sleep

Sleep is made up of specific stages with distinctive characteristics of eye movement and muscle tension that are prompted by natural cycles of brain activity. These sleep stages can be identified through the use of an electro-encephalograph (EEG), which measures brain wave patterns during a sleep study (polysomnogram). The two broad categories of sleep include non–rapid eye movement (NREM) sleep and rapid eye movement (REM) sleep.

NREM sleep is composed of four different levels, or stages. Each stage is characterized by different combinations of brain waves, eye movements, and degrees of reduced but not absent muscle tension.

Stage 1 sleep is the beginning of the sleep cycle. When the light is off and you close your eyes, your brain waves slow as does your breathing and heart rate. Your muscles start to relax. This sleep stage is the transition from wakefulness to light sleep. If someone wakes you up from Stage 1 sleep, you may not even believe you were really asleep. Stage 1 sleep usually makes up about 5 percent of total sleep time.

Stage 2 sleep is slightly deeper than Stage 1 sleep, but it is still a stage from which you can awaken easily. Here you may feel like you are falling (you may even wake up) and you become less and less aware of your environment. Stage 2 sleep typically accounts for 40 to 50 percent of total sleep time.

Stages 3 and 4 sleep (deep sleep or delta sleep) account for 20 percent of total sleep time in young adults. Older adults spend about 10 to 15 percent of total sleep time in this sleep stage, depending on their medical conditions and medications. Delta sleep is the deepest level of NREM sleep and usually occurs during the first third of the night. In these stages of sleep, blood pressure drops more, muscles become more relaxed, and your blood flow decreases. Growth hormone is secreted by your pituitary gland in the deep-sleep stage. During this stage, your body heals itself and

SLEEP STAGES FOR AVERAGE ADULTS

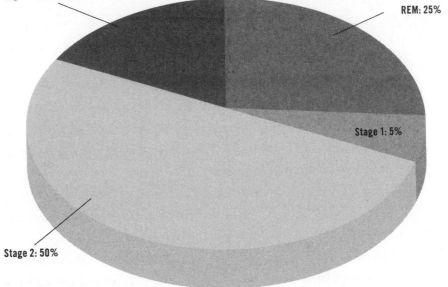

Stages 3 and 4: 20%

REM: 25%

Stage 1: 5%

Stage 2: 50%

you experience repair and tissue regeneration; *this is the physical restoration stage of sleep.* When you get enough delta or deep sleep, you awake refreshed and ready to meet the day just like a bear after a long winter.

REM sleep takes place mostly during the last third of your night's sleep and usually makes up 25 percent of your sleep time, though this may decrease with age. During REM sleep, there are small, variable-speed brain waves; rapid eye movements like those that occur during eyes-open wakefulness; and no muscle tension. All voluntary muscles are paralyzed, but your heart and the muscles that power your lungs and eyes remain active during REM sleep. It's during this stage that you restore your nervous system, process information, and store memories. Although dreams can occur in any sleep stage, you have your most vivid dreams during REM sleep. If you are awakened from REM sleep, you can recall vivid imagery. *This is the mental restoration stage of sleep.* When you get enough REM sleep, you think more quickly and creatively and are able to organize your thoughts better.

SLEEP DIET FACT: You cannot lose weight if your biological clock is off rhythm.

After you fall asleep, a normal sleep cycle takes you from light sleep into deep sleep and then back to light sleep and then on to REM sleep. After REM sleep, your body awakens briefly and then returns to Stage 1 sleep to repeat the process. Throughout the night, you cycle through the sleep stages, with REM sleep increasing in length with each cycle and deep sleep decreasing toward morning. *To be fully renewed and feel refreshed in the morning, you need ample amounts of each type of sleep.*

Each sleep cycle—one complete run through all the stages—lasts about 90 minutes. For sleep to be restorative, you need several complete sleep cycles every night; most people require four to five complete cycles. Many of my patients feel powerful and productive after 7.5 hours of sleep, or five 90-minute sleep cycles; others claim to be at their best with more or less sleep. This depends upon the length of their personal sleep cycles.

Sleep Rhythm and Sleep Drive

Your sleep and its daily relationship with wakefulness are controlled by two systems[1]:

1. **Your biological clock,** or **circadian rhythm,** which is the waxing and waning biochemical cycle that repeats roughly every 24 hours and governs sleep-wake times, hunger, body temperature, hormone release, and other subtle rhythms that mesh with the 24-hour day.

2. **Your sleep drive (the need for sleep)** dictates the amount and intensity of sleep you need based on how long you've been awake. Think of your sleep drive like hunger; it builds throughout the day until it is satisfied.

Morning Lark or Night Owl?

Everyone's circadian clock, or sleep pacemaker, ticks at a slightly different rate. You probably have some idea of whether you are an early bird or night owl. Your sleep-wake schedule is influenced by your personal body clock, and early birds have a different circadian cycle than night owls.

SLEEP 101

EARLY BIRD OR NIGHT OWL?

In some cases I see people who force themselves to wake up and go to sleep at certain times, especially if work and social activities dictate their schedules and boundaries. Allowing your social, family, and work lives to run your sleep-wake schedule instead of the opposite—especially when these two schedules conflict—is a common cause of many sleep problems. To compromise, find out what your body wants and then take that into consideration as you try to find balance by making some adjustments to both your sleep-wake schedule and the commitments you have during the day.

Review the list below to see which reflects you best.

	EARLY BIRD	NIGHT OWL
I feel alert . . .	In the early morning	Late in the evening
I feel the sleepiest . . .	In the early evening	Past midnight
I enjoy waking up . . .	At 6 a.m. or earlier	At 8 a.m. or later
I have the most energy . . .	A few hours after waking	A few hours before bed

For example, if you are a night owl who needs to be at work by 8:30 a.m., instead of getting up at 6:30 a.m. to get ready, try moving that time to 6:45 a.m. and then 7:00 a.m. More sleep time will make a big difference. Another quick tip: Never use the snooze button; all this does is allow you to go back into light, unrefreshing sleep, which does little good.

We believe that there are two body clocks—one that is set by the outer cues of light and darkness and a neurological clock that follows a schedule set by the brain.[2] When these two clocks aren't on the same schedule and compete with one another, you feel out of sorts, as you do when you have jet lag, for example, or when you change your work schedule.

Melatonin Sets the Brain's Biological Clock

The hormone most closely linked with the circadian system is melatonin, which is made by the pineal gland, in the center of the brain. Along with sunlight, the body's primary timekeeper, melatonin helps to set the brain's biological clock. During the biological night, melatonin is secreted, the body temperature lowers, and sleep propensity increases.

Supplemental melatonin is available over the counter, without a prescription. But I do not recommend IT. Remember, melatonin is a hormone, not a vitamin or mineral, and while "natural" it is rarely used correctly and could be dangerous.

Richard Wurtman, MD, and colleagues from MIT have discovered that melatonin supplementation of between 0.3 and 1 milligram will give you an effective level of melatonin for sleep regulation.[3] Most OTC melatonin is in an overdose pill, and taking too much, especially of a hormone, can have some serious side effects. Since it is not regulated by the FDA, producers are not held to specific purity standards during manufacture, nor is the dosage regulated, which can be dangerous. Remember: Melatonin is a circadian clock regulator, not a sleeping pill. If you use it, do so only under the care of a sleep specialist, and only if your biological clock needs a temporary adjustment. Also, it is not something I recommend for use by children of any age. Melatonin has documented effects on the regulation of ovarian function—at high dosages, it has been used as a contraceptive—and we have no idea what effects it could have on a young reproductive system.

In some sleep research studies, scientists report that subjects who take melatonin an hour before bedtime fall asleep more quickly and sleep longer than those given a placebo. Yet all an over-the-counter melatonin supplement does is change the timing of the presence of melatonin in the sleep system. If you went into a dark room when your core body temperature was dropping, the pineal gland would likely produce enough melatonin to get you to sleep. It is incredibly rare to have a melatonin deficiency, and taking too much of a supplement at the wrong time could make you very sleepy when you need to be wide awake!

Sleep Rhythms and Sleep Drive

Your sleep quality or intensity is reflected by:

- The amount of delta or deep sleep (Stages 3 and 4) you get each night
- Your ability to stay continuously asleep
- The overall number of minutes of sleep
- Whether or not you sleep at the right times in your circadian cycle

When all of these factors come together, you have great sleep quality. But when even one of these areas is out of sync, your sleep quality declines rapidly. What are some other factors that can affect your sleep quality? The triggers of what I call *disordered sleep.*

SLEEP 101

SLEEPING PILLS ARE NOT THE NEW DIET PILL

Can Ambien make me thin? This is a question I have gotten before so let's get straight to the heart of the matter. Sleeping pills are not diet pills. Sleeping pills are controlled substances that should be taken only under the supervision of your prescribing doctor. (Never take someone else's pills.) Could the side effect from any sleep treatment—where your sleep quality and quantity is improved—be weight loss? Absolutely. But sleeping pills may only improve the quantity or duration of your sleep and may not provide the overall long term improvement in sleep quality that you may need.

Sleep Disorder versus Disordered Sleep

SLEEP DIET FACT: You should awaken feeling relatively refreshed and remain alert throughout the day—every day.

Let's get something straight: *You are not supposed to be sleepy during the day if you are getting a sufficient quantity and quality of sleep at night.* If you are asleep literally before your head hits the pillow, this is a good sign that you are not getting enough sleep.

Understanding Sleep Disorders

The distinction between a sleep disorder and what I call disordered sleep is important. Sleep disorders are formal syndromes with defined criteria and recur with some regularity. They can be primary sleep disorders, which cannot be attributed to other conditions, or secondary sleep disorders that arise due to an underlying physical or mental condition. For example, *restless legs syndrome,* in which a creeping, crawling sensation in the legs and sometimes in the arms creates an irresistible urge to move, is a *primary sleep disorder. Insomnia,* which is characterized by difficulty in falling or staying asleep or by awakening too early, can be a *secondary sleep disorder.* This is because it is often linked to depression or some other underlying physiological cause that warrants treatment. Often, a primary sleep disorder can give rise to a secondary sleep disorder. For example, someone who has restless legs syndrome could develop insomnia as a result of his or her chronic inability to sleep soundly. In such cases, treating the symptoms of the primary sleep disorder often improves the symptoms of other sleep disorders.

Once a disorder has been identified, the goal is to systematically develop a therapy to either avert the symptoms associated with it or cure the underlying problem. There are about 88 recognized sleep disorders, the best known of which are insomnia, sleep apnea, narcolepsy, and restless legs syndrome. (See below for more on sleep disorders.) But here's what I want you to remember:

SLEEP DIET FACT: You cannot lose weight when you have an untreated sleep disorder.

If you think you are suffering from a sleep disorder, then you should seek the counsel of a qualified sleep specialist as soon as possible. To find one, go to www.sleepcenters.org.

Could You Have a Sleep Disorder?

If you get 7 to 8 hours of sleep and still feel as if you didn't sleep well, you could have a sleep disorder.[4] While many sleep problems arise from poor sleep hygiene, too much caffeine, PMS, or daily stress, a sleep disorder is a *formal medical diagnosis* that needs the attention of a sleep specialist. Left untreated, sleep disorders can result in hypertension, heart disease, stroke, depression, diabetes, and other chronic diseases, even death. There are about 88 recognized sleep disorders. Some of the more common ones for women include:

- **Insomnia**—This is disruption of the sleep cycle caused by difficulty getting to sleep, difficulty staying asleep, or awakening too early. Insomnia is the most common sleep problem, and women are more likely than men to report it.[5]

- **Sleep apnea**—This potentially life-threatening problem causes a person to stop breathing as a result of relaxed or excessive tissue blocking the airway. One out of 50 middle-aged women has sleep apnea; being overweight, having a thick neck, or having gone through menopause makes women much more likely to develop it.[6] Long-term sleep deprivation from sleep disorders such as apnea has been implicated in high blood pressure, heart attack, and stroke. See the "Sleep Alert!," opposite, for symptoms of sleep apnea.

- **Restless legs syndrome**—This is a creeping, crawling sensation in the legs (and sometimes the arms) that creates an irresistible urge to move. Studies show that restless legs syndrome (RLS) is mainly due to an iron deficiency. Having a blood ferritin level of less than 60 nanograms per milliliter (determined by a lab test) can give rise to the symptoms of RLS. It is more common in pregnant women (one in four of them are affected) and occurs during the last trimester of pregnancy. In addition, RLS has a genetic component and often runs in families. About 40 percent of those who are diagnosed with this sleep disorder have symptoms before age 20.[7, 8, 9]

- **Periodic limb movements in sleep**—Characterized by sudden and uncontrollable twitching or jerking of the arms or legs every 10 to 60 seconds during sleep and that in many cases will wake you from sleep, this condition makes sound sleep difficult. It is more common in women and occurs in up to 34 percent of those over 60 years old.[10]

If any of these descriptions sound like things you experience, talk to your doctor. You may need a full evaluation by a sleep specialist.

!SLEEP !ALERT

If you feel that you have any of the following signs and symptoms of sleep apnea, speak to your doctor immediately.

- Snoring
- Observed apnea episodes (when you stop breathing during sleep)
- Morning headaches and dry mouth
- Daytime sleepiness after adequate sleep of 7 to 9 hours
- Mood swings or depression

A New Concept: Disordered Sleep

"Disordered sleep" means any sleep problem that is not a bona fide sleep disorder. Your sleep symptoms might not quite meet the sleep disorder criteria based on severity or frequency, or there might be an external factor that's affecting your sleep, such as a cat in your bed or too much heat in the room or a bad mattress or pillow, but they result in less or lower-quality sleep. Disordered sleep also reflects the value you place (or don't place) on sleep.

For the vast majority of people, disordered sleep is a major problem. In fact, sleep problems often occur as the result of poor sleep hygiene—bad habits that don't support a good sleep experience. Thus, sometimes disordered sleep leads to a sleep disorder. Such habits encompass a range of practices and environmental factors, many of which you can control, including:

- Smoking or drinking alcoholic or caffeinated beverages
- Exercising vigorously or eating a large meal before bed
- Experiencing jet lag from travel across time zones
- Dealing with psychological stressors such as deadlines, exams, marital conflict, or job crises

All of these can impair your ability to fall asleep or stay asleep. Designing and staying with a good sleep hygiene regimen, which you will do on *The Sleep Doctor's Diet Plan,* should alleviate these types of problems, or at least give you a disciplined way to handle them so they only minimally affect your sleep.

A Quick Summary

At this point you should have a better understanding of what sleep is from a physiological standpoint. You now know:

1. Sleep is made up of five identifiable stages (Stages 1, 2, 3, 4, and REM).
   a. Stages 3 and 4 are physically restorative sleep.
   b. REM is mentally restorative sleep.

2. There is a circadian rhythm to sleep that follows a roughly 24-hour cycle.

3. There is a biological drive to make you sleep that is similar to the hunger drive.

4. You are either an early bird or a night owl.

5. Melatonin is a hormone produced in the brain that helps regulate your circadian rhythm, and OTC melatonin supplements can be dangerous.

6. The average sleep cycle is 90 minutes long, and the average person has four to five cycles each night.

7. Sleep quality is determined by several factors.

8. There is a difference between a *sleep disorder* and *disordered sleep.*

In the next chapter, I'll explain how any or all of these sleep disruptions can wreak havoc on your body's ability to regulate your weight and keep your metabolism working efficiently.

3

The Sleep/Metabolism
Matrix

Some of the factors contributing to weight loss through better sleep—having more energy for exercising, having less need for the sugary, temporarily energy-boosting snacks that lead to weight gain—are rather obvious and quite easy to understand. But the connection between sleep and weight goes far beyond these simple connections. The latest science shows that our metabolic rate appears to change based not only on our age, gender, and medical issues, but also on how well (or how poorly) we sleep. The physiological functions that influence eating, energy balance, and metabolism are strongly tied to circadian rhythms (see page 29) and sleep. In other words, disrupting your biological clock can have important metabolic consequences that affect your weight for months or years to come.[1] Even in very lean individuals, experiments have shown that short-term sleep restriction affects glucose tolerance and cortisol and growth hormone secretion.[2]

It's been well established that obesity is on the rise in the United States, but it's not solely because of dietary habits, genetics, and less physical activity. There seem to be environmental, social, and behavioral influences that promote overeating and inactivity. Ironically, these same factors also influence your sleep.

One of the markers for body fat that's used by many doctors today is a calculation using your weight and height that measures what's called the *body mass index (BMI)*. Under this system, an adult who has a BMI of between 25 and 29.9 is considered overweight; an adult with a BMI of 30 or higher is considered obese. To calculate your own BMI, go to www.nhlbisupport.com/bmi.

While the BMI is used by many health care practitioners to determine if patients are overweight or obese, *it can be misleading in some adults*, especially men and women who have large frames or an abundance of muscle. Even though these men and women may have BMIs of higher than 25, they might not have excessive body fat. Talk to your doctor about your weight to see if you are at risk for obesity.

Less-Sleep Trend Parallels Obesity Epidemic

As we saw in the chart on page 11, the rise in obesity parallels with uncanny accuracy a corresponding decrease in sleep hours over the very same time frame. It's quite disturbing to me to see the

SLEEP DIET FACT: Sleep loss leads to either an increase in calories taken in or a decrease in calories burned off.

correspondence between the obesity rate of more than 35 percent of adults in the United States and the least sleep time per night in history of 6.5 hours.

Of course, there are other factors at play, including sedentary lifestyles, genetics, and chronic overeating. Still, groundbreaking research continues to link sleeping less with being overweight or obese. In fact, epidemiologic studies from Spain, Japan, and the United States show an interesting relationship between BMI and sleep in women. Women who had the lowest, healthiest BMIs (20 to 25) spent on average 7.7 hours in bed per night.[3] In addition, a few studies link *too much sleep* to overweight or obesity.

AVERAGE NIGHTLY SLEEP AND BODY MASS INDEX IN WOMEN[4]

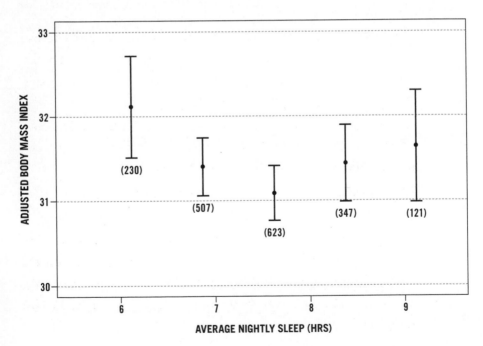

Why Does Too Little Sleep Seem to Lead to Weight Gain?

Right now, we know several reasons why sleep loss results in added weight—possibly even obesity.

- People who sleep less take in more calories.
  - **When you are sleep deprived, your body does not get rid of the food you eat, so it is stored as fat.** This occurs because of an alteration in your body's glucose metabolism.
  - **When you are sleep deprived, there is an increase in your appetite.** This increase occurs because of an imbalance in your hormone levels.
  - **When you are sleep deprived, you have more time to eat** (generally snacks).
- People who sleep less burn fewer calories.
  - **With sleep loss, there is a decrease in your body's ability to use calories (reducing your energy expenditure).** Although the findings are not conclusive, studies continue to show a clear link between sleep loss and how people burn calories.
  - **A few studies show that REM sleep burns more calories than any of the other sleep stages.** And if your sleep is shortened, you are likely losing important REM sleep![5]
- People who sleep less lose less fat if they do lose weight.
  - Recently, scientists confirmed that when dieters got plenty of sleep (8.5 hours), they lost the same amount of weight as when they slept less. *However, when dieters got adequate sleep, the weight they lost was fat.* When they slept less (only 5.5 hours), they lost lean body mass—plus they claimed to be hungrier.[6]

Sugar, Aw . . . Honey, Honey!

To understand why changes in glucose metabolism occur, we have to go back to basic physiology. Your body is constantly trying to balance out the glucose in your system. Remember, glucose (a simple sugar) is one of the basic building blocks of every food that you eat. Your body breaks down food into glucose to use as energy. Having too much glucose in your system, a condition called hyperglycemia (high blood sugar), is a major problem for people with diabetes, and it can have big consequences for your health. Symptoms of hyperglycemia include frequent urination, increased thirst, and high levels of sugar in the urine. When you have too little glucose in your system, a condition called hypoglycemia or low blood sugar, you have symptoms such as dizziness, shakiness, sweating, hunger, headache, paleness, sudden moodiness for no apparent reason, clumsiness, seizure, and inattentiveness.[7]

"Homeostasis," or balance, is achieved when the liver produces glucose from food and then the tissues of your body use the right amount of it. Your muscles and fat use the glucose with the help of insulin secreted by the pancreas. Organs such as the brain use the glucose without the help of insulin.

Sleep loss also affects the ability to process foods such as carbohydrates, which ultimately leads to increased blood glucose (blood sugar). As your blood sugar level rises, your pancreas overproduces insulin. This results in the storage of excess body fat and possible development of type 2 diabetes, which is defined as a chronically elevated level of glucose in the blood. Type 2 diabetes is the most common form of diabetes, affecting 90 to 95 percent of the 24 million people with diabetes in the United States today.[8] Another 57 million Americans over age 20 are considered prediabetic, having blood glucose levels that are chronically higher than normal, but not as high as those in people with diabetes.

GLUCOSE SEESAW: PRODUCTION BY LIVER VERSUS USE BY TISSUES

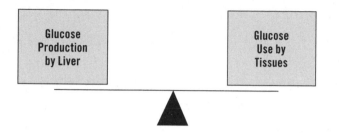

The balance of glucose production and use changes throughout the day and night as one of your circadian rhythms. Your body's glucose utilization rate is higher in the morning than in the evening. In the first half of the night, you use glucose more slowly because your body doesn't require as much of it during deep sleep (Stages 3 and 4), when it rests and heals.

However, glucose metabolism starts to increase in the second half of the night when you enter REM sleep. And amazingly, *the better you sleep, the more calories you burn*. The longer you sleep, the more REM sleep you get, so you will burn more calories if you sleep longer.[9] However, as we have seen with the BMI index, there is a happy medium. Those who sleep *too long* have slower metabolisms because they stay in bed instead of expending energy!

Sleep Deprived = More Stored Fat

When your body is even slightly sleep deprived, three things happen. First, you hold on to glucose longer. Sleep deprivation also causes your body to use this glucose less efficiently. Finally, when you are sleep deprived, your body's ability to create insulin quickly when you eat food is reduced. In summary, if your body is even partially sleep deprived, the food you eat is not burned by your metabolism as quickly or efficiently. *The result? The food is stored as fat!*

How Less Sleep Results in Hormone Havoc

SLEEP DIET FACT: At least four hormones that are affected by sleep influence weight gain—ghrelin, leptin, cortisol, and growth hormone.

I like to think of hormones as messengers connecting various systems and command centers of the body; they get produced in one part of the body by tissues and glands such as the thyroid, adrenals, and pituitary and then pass into the bloodstream for delivery to distant organs and tissues, where they act to modify structures and functions.

Did you know that your appetite is regulated by signals your hormones send to your brain? There is a specific place in the brain—the arcuate nucleus of the hypothalamus—that controls the on/off switch for appetite. This tiny part of the brain also controls body temperature, thirst, fatigue, and most circadian rhythms.

Hormones act like traffic signs and signals by telling your body what to do and when and making sure its machinery runs smoothly and maintains homeostasis, or balance. Hormones are used by all organ systems, and *their proper balance relies on sleep.* Much of how you *feel*—tired, ravenous, full, excited, thirsty, hot, cold, stressed out—is related to the secretion of hormones and their impacts on your mind and body. There are many hormones that are affected by sleep and that, in turn, affect weight, but the basic ones involved are leptin, ghrelin, cortisol, and growth hormone.

The Stop and Go Appetite Hormones

SLEEP DIET FACT: Ghrelin and leptin hold the remote control for your hunger and appetite.

Two hormones, ghrelin and leptin, hold the remote control for your appetite. Ghrelin is the green light that says, "Go get some food!" Leptin is the red light that says, "Stop eating now!"

Ghrelin is secreted by your stomach when it's empty, increasing your appetite. It sends a message to your brain that says, "I'm hungry. Feed me."

When your stomach is full, leptin, which is secreted by fat cells, sends a message to your brain that says, "Stop eating. I'm done." This appetite hormone regulates food intake, energy expenditure, and body weight. Leptin decreases appetite by causing you to feel full and increases energy output by telling you that you have fuel you can burn. Scientists believe that people who are obese may have a problem with the receptors for leptin in their brains, so their appetites do not respond when this hormone says, "Stop eating now." In some cases, they even may be getting the opposite message—"Keep eating"—from leptin. But how do these two appetite hormones relate to sleep?

Poor sleep lowers the level of leptin (the "stop" hormone) and boosts the production of ghrelin (the "go" hormone), resulting in your feeling hungrier. One key study at the University of Chicago showed that when healthy men were allowed just 4 hours of sleep a night for 2 nights, they averaged an 18 percent drop in leptin and a 28 percent increase in ghrelin.[10] These sleep-deprived participants perceived an average 24 percent increase in their hunger and a 23 percent increase in their appetite—particularly for high-calorie and high-carb foods. "Hunger"—the sensation that precedes eating—is the feeling of wanting to eat, and "appetite" is the physical need to eat until full. When your brain doesn't get the message that you are full, you keep eating and eating . . . and eating.

With normal sleep, there are small initial rises in leptin and ghrelin at night. During the second half of the night, ghrelin decreases. However, comprehensive research shows that partial sleep deprivation (*sleeping less than about 6.5 hours*) causes the level of leptin to be lower and the level of ghrelin to be higher during the day—even when the body should be sending signals to say that it has had enough food.[11]

The study showed that total sleep time was negatively correlated with the circulating level of ghrelin. Therefore, the less sleep a person got, the more ghrelin he or she produced. The accuracy of the brain's assessment of whether it needs more energy (food) is questionable when a person is sleep deprived.[12]

Thus, when you are sleep deprived, a signal may be sent to your brain to ask for *more food* even when your stomach is full!

Cortisol, the Stress Hormone

Another chemical that can increase your appetite is cortisol, a naturally occurring hormone that helps to regulate glucose. This hormone causes your body to break down muscles for energy and store excess calories as fat. And, as you might have guessed, you want to control your level of cortisol if you are trying to lose weight.

Problem is, *you can't control your level of cortisol without getting enough sleep.* Lack of sleep increases cortisol production, making you store fat and burn muscle. A high cortisol level also *increases your appetite!* In other words, poor sleep does the exact opposite of what you are trying to accomplish. Not surprisingly, your cortisol level is highest early in the morning while you are still sleeping and during periods of high stress, and lowest in the early stages of deep sleep. Some fat-burning supplements allege that they can combat the effects of cortisol. But a good night's sleep is the far better, more effective remedy. As you'll learn later in this book, diet supplements that contain stimulants can hinder sound sleep and ultimately work against your weight-loss goals.

Stress More, Weigh More

Cortisol is produced by the adrenal glands, the primary mission of which is to produce a hormone that converts stored energy into usable energy. When you find yourself in a threatening situation, the brain activates these glands to release cortisol, which literally puts energy in your personal fuel tank in the form of blood glucose.

When you have an acute emergency or one that lasts for a short time—a few hours, perhaps even a couple of days—usually no permanent physical damage is done. Your heart rate and blood pressure increase, and the alarm neurotransmitter, adrenaline (which is also produced by the adrenal glands), floods your body, making your heart beat faster and increasing the bloodflow to your muscles and intestines.

When stress is present for days or weeks, it is called *chronic stress*. In response to it, the adrenal glands keep pouring out cortisol, and problems arise. The elevated cortisol level makes you burn up your body's readily available resource (glucose in the blood) for energy until there is no more available. Then, instead of drawing upon stored energy (fat), your body begins to break down muscle and other tissues to keep going. So a high cortisol level leads to the breakdown of muscle and other tissues—*but not of fat.* In addition, long-term cortisol overproduction because of chronic stress inhibits sleep, which increases your appetite. Remember that during sleep is when your primary neurotransmitters get replenished. Without this replenishment, you feel fatigued, achy, and depressed.

Another problem with chronic stress is that cortisol increases the desire for carbohydrates by increasing the production of neuropeptide Y, a neurotransmitter found in the brain. Sarah Leibowitz, PhD, of Rockefeller University, found that neuropeptide Y stimulates eating, particularly of carbohydrates. Neuropeptide Y has its greatest effect on appetite early in the day, after the overnight fast, and its level is increased after any period of deprivation—including dieting.[13]

So, it is not surprising that dieters and people under stress reach for high-carbohydrate foods that pack on the pounds, such as breads, sweets, pasta, and cereals.

If you do not have a healthy way of coping with chronic stress, your constant exposure to stress hormones will eventually cause your body to become overloaded. When you're stressed out for a long period of time, it can result in a dramatic decline in both your physical and mental health and a possible incline in your weight.

Stress, Sleep Loss, and Belly Fat

When cortisol levels remain high from chronic stress and sleep loss, the associated accumulation of abdominal fat (also called belly fat and visceral fat) expands the waistline and results in an apple-shaped body.[14] We're now learning that people with apple-shaped bodies have an increased blood level of a proinflammatory marker called C-reactive protein that indicates that they're at greater risk for diabetes and cardiovascular disease. Some findings indicate that greater girth is more closely associated with inflammation than obesity concentrated in other parts of the body.[15]

C-reactive protein is produced by the liver only during episodes of acute inflammation. It is highly correlated with obesity, cardiovascular diseases, diabetes, and cancers. The good news is that weight loss is associated with a *significant decrease in proinflammatory markers* like C-reactive protein, as well as decreases in LDL ("bad") cholesterol and triglyceride levels, blood pressure, and fasting blood glucose level.[16]

During our younger years, when cortisol secretion is stimulated by stress, a feedback mechanism based in the hypothalamus shuts the cortisol off. As we get older, however, this feedback loop does not work so well, and our ability to manage the stress response is compromised. Stress interferes with weight loss and disrupts normal sleep by interfering with the sleep cycle.

Losing sleep also boosts the secretion of cortisol, making us feel hungrier and have unnecessary cravings.

"Stressed" Is "Desserts" Spelled Backward

Studies show that stress and the associated sleep loss do two things to affect your weight.[17]

1. **Stress and sleep loss make you feel hungry even if you are full.** That's because losing sleep increases the secretion of cortisol, the stress hormone that regulates your appetite. As a result, when you get poor sleep or not enough sleep, you feel ravenous even when you've eaten plenty of food.

2. **Stress and sleep loss increase fat storage.** Sleep loss interferes with the body's ability to metabolize carbohydrates. This interference can lead to a high blood glucose level. High blood sugar triggers the overproduction of insulin, which then leads to the storage of body fat and a condition called *insulin resistance.*

STRESS AND SLEEP HORMONES

HORMONE	WHAT IT'S SUPPOSED TO DO	WHAT IT DOES WHEN YOU'RE STRESSED	WHAT IT DOES WHEN YOU'RE SLEEP DEPRIVED
CORTISOL (THE STRESS HORMONE)	Increases your blood sugar; helps you metabolize fat, protein, and carbohydrates; suppresses your immune system	Increases its blood level to give you energy; increases your appetite; over time, damages your body	Increases your appetite; decreases your immune function
SEROTONIN (A NEUROTRANSMITTER)	Helps transmit messages along your nerve pathways	Becomes depleted, causing burnout	Makes you want to eat simple sugars
GHRELIN (THE "GO" HORMONE)	Tells you to eat more	Increases its production	Increases your appetite
LEPTIN (THE "STOP" HORMONE)	Tells you to stop eating	Decreases its production	Makes you feel less full than you really are
INSULIN	Helps regulate your blood sugar level	Decreases its production	Increases your fat stores

Wait! Don't Forget about Growth Hormone

Poor sleep also deprives the body of adequate growth hormone (GH). GH is a powerful antiobesity hormone that decreases the rate at which your cells utilize carbohydrates and increases the rate at which they use fats (all good for weight loss!). We now know that as deep-sleep time decreases, so does the secretion of GH. In addition, by the time a person is 35, GH production can have decreased by as much as 75 percent due to aging. And sleep deprivation could make this worse.

As soon as you hit deep sleep, about 20 to 30 minutes after you first close your eyes and then again during each sleep cycle, your pituitary gland starts to release high levels of GH—the most it will secrete at any point in the day. Without that sleep, your level of GH is significantly reduced, negatively affecting your proportion of fat to muscle. Over time, a chronically low GH level is associated with more fat and less lean muscle.

If you're finding it hard to keep these hormones—leptin, ghrelin, cortisol, and growth hormone—straight, don't worry; the chart below will guide you.

HORMONE	WHAT SLEEP LOSS DOES TO IT
LEPTIN	Reduces it, so you eat more because there is nothing telling you to "stop"
GHRELIN	Increases it, so you eat more because it says "go"
CORTISOL	Increases it, so you eat more
GROWTH HORMONE	Reduces it, so you store more glucose as fat

Sleep Loss and Snacks

When you are sleep deprived, do you find that you snack more? Several recent studies have shown that people who are sleep deprived seek extra calories in the form of snack foods. In one study published in the *American Journal of Clinical Nutrition*,[18] researchers found that when volunteers had slept only 5.5 hours, they ate their normal amounts at mealtimes, *but their snack intake increased dramatically.* On average, these people ate about *1,000 calories in snacks* (65 percent of them carbohydrates), all of it *between 11 p.m. and 7 a.m.!*

Sleep Loss and Energy Expenditure

The amount of energy the body uses over a given time period is called its energy expenditure, and it is the sum of several different components.

- **Your resting metabolic rate,** which uses up about 60 percent of your energy
- **The thermic effect of food** (the energy used to digest, absorb, metabolize, and store food), which accounts for about 10 percent of your energy expenditure
- **The energy you burn in activity** (everything you do), which requires about 30 percent of your energy

Currently, there's not enough research to conclusively link weight gain with the decrease in energy expenditure that is related to sleep loss. But there are some interesting signs that point in that direction.

- In animal studies, increased ghrelin (the "go" hormone) increases food intake and decreases motor activity[19]
- Sleep deprivation decreases the motivation to exercise[20]
- People with sleep disorders have significantly reduced levels of physical activity[21]

Thus, the research suggests that *sleep loss results in decreased physical activity and in weight gain.* Still, we cannot say for sure that there are not other factors influencing energy expenditure.

Ultimately it seems likely, as well as logical, that your body's ability to use glucose and your hormones' effects on your appetite and fat storage are related to both sleep loss and weight gain.

Sabotage Your Diet with Sleep Loss

Sleep loss, in a sense, disconnects your brain from your stomach. With sleep loss, eating becomes an unconscious act, and you also have a hard time controlling *what* you eat. The Chicago study mentioned earlier in this chapter found that the volunteers' appetites for calorie-dense, high-carbohydrate foods like sweets, salty snacks, and starchy foods *increased by 33 to 45 percent when they slept only 4 hours a night.* This translates into two strikes against you when you get too little sleep.

1. Sleep loss tricks your body into believing it is hungry when it's not.
2. Sleep loss makes you crave foods that can sabotage a healthy diet. You'll want the cake and ice cream instead of the bowl of fruit and yogurt. And you won't be able to stop eating as easily. (This study was not a fluke.)

Less Sleep, More Sweets

Other studies have found that in people of normal weight, leptin decreases the perception of a sweet taste, making sweet foods less appealing. Reduced leptin makes people who are overweight and obese continue to taste the sweetness. Since loss of sleep causes the body to produce less leptin, *if you are overweight and sleep deprived, your appetite will seem to never be satisfied, and everything you stuff in your mouth will taste great!*

All of these findings point to the same conclusion: *Sleep loss results in weight gain.* Even though the sleep/obesity link is complicated, its existence is substantiated by the latest scientific studies, and the medical community is beginning to recognize the critical role proper sleep plays in weight regulation.

But there is much more. The unique aspects of being a woman have a dramatic effect on your ability to get good-quality sleep. In the next chapter, I will tell you how your menstrual cycle, pregnancy, and menopause are guaranteed sleep disrupters, and I'll give you some sleep tips to use during these times.

4

The Unique
Sleep Challenges
of Women

G etting good sleep is hard for many people today. But you're a woman, so it can be even harder for you! Here's extra information you need to know.

About 6 years ago, Claire, a senior researcher for a pharmaceutical company in California, started having sleep problems. Then 34, she had given birth to her second child a year earlier.

Claire simply couldn't sleep. She thought she had tried everything—from eliminating caffeine in her diet, to exercising in the early morning hours, to taking over-the-counter herbal sleep supplements—all to no avail. Over several months, Claire's sleep debt (her accumulated missed sleep) increased tremendously, interfering with her ability to manage her difficult research assignments. She talked to her ob/gyn, who had few answers other than prescription sleep aids, but Claire didn't want to go that route. She wanted a natural solution to her problems.

Claire realized that she needed to understand sleep and what was keeping her from sleeping. Her career, income, health, and ability to manage her active family all depended upon her finding ways to sleep well.

While working with Claire, I realized that normal hormonal fluctuations associated with her menstrual cycle were having a dramatic effect on her sleep. I educated her about the particular phases of the menstrual cycle and how the stages of sleep were being adversely affected by the changing levels of estrogen and progesterone, and we also talked a good bit about rescheduling her busy life.

I suggested Claire keep a *Sleep Diary*. In a simple notebook, she wrote down the following.

1. The time she went to bed
2. The time she thought she fell asleep
3. The number of times she woke up during the night
4. The time she woke up for the day
5. Her intake of caffeine, alcohol, and nicotine
6. Her use of over-the-counter (OTC) medicines such as Tylenol PM or similar formulations that can impact sleep
7. A subjective rating of her sleep from 1 to 5 (1 is poor; 5 is great)

Using the Sleep Diary as a guide, I asked Claire to map her monthly sleep schedule.

At her next visit, Claire noted that she needed more sleep during the week of her period, and she agreed to get the kids to bed earlier and change her own bedtime during that week. Claire had major food cravings for high-fat, high-sugar foods like homemade chocolate chip cookies and candy bars in the week before her period. These cravings usually came on in the evenings, and many of these foods disturbed her sleep and added a few pounds to her frame. I gave her a list of sleep-promoting foods, including whole grain bagels, cereals, and crackers, that boost the level of serotonin, a naturally occurring brain chemical that is calming and reduces anxiety. In addition, I asked Claire to make sure she was sleeping well before her period, so the cravings would not be intensified.

Within a month, Claire had conquered many of her sleep issues. In fact, she lost 4 pounds without changing her diet (except for making better bedtime snack choices). Having a greater understanding of how female hormonal fluctuations affected her sleep each month fully armed her to work with her body to change her sleep habits and be rewarded with better sleep.

Chances are that if you are female, you have experienced major sleep issues like Claire's. Younger women tell me that their sleep is interrupted by PMS symptoms and menstruation. Pregnant women can barely wake up because of the surge of sleep-inducing progesterone their bodies release, or they are so uncomfortable because of the pregnancy that they cannot sleep. And caring for the needs of a newborn during the postpartum period puts sleep on the back burner for many new moms. And with the decline of estrogen at menopause, women at midlife complain about hot flashes and night sweats that disrupt their sleep and ruin their nights. According to the National Sleep Foundation, approximately 61 percent of postmenopausal women have sleep problems.[1] *Fortunately, there are simple answers to many of these complaints, as you will read in this chapter!*

Women's Sleep Is Different from Men's

Until recently, much of the research on and treatment and understanding of sleep were based on studies that focused on men, even though *women report far more sleep problems than men do.*[2] The media and the population in general have received too little medical information on women and sleep, particularly about sleep problems women have at different ages and stages in life[3] and how they can get good-quality sleep each night.

The fact is, women have more problems sleeping than men do for two primary reasons: *hormones* and *aging*.

Hormones Wreak Havoc

Women have more problems falling asleep and staying asleep than men do and are also more likely to have daytime sleepiness. Women have more sleep disruptions during the premenstrual and menstrual times of the month—including difficulty getting to sleep, nighttime awakenings, sleep disturbances, and vivid dreams.[4,5]

But why do these sleep disruptions occur? Your hormones. While the hormone estrogen, which is present in both sexes but more abundant in women, increases REM sleep, the female hormone progesterone, which rises at midcycle, after ovulation, causes feelings of fatigue and drowsiness. When menstruation begins and the progesterone level begins to fall, women have greater difficulties falling asleep and often experience poor sleep quality for a few days. As a woman's cycle begins again, normal sleep (if not good sleep) usually returns. Other consequences women must contend with include:

- **Changes in the rhythm of body temperature** throughout the menstrual cycle that affect sleep. Your sleep pattern seems to closely follow changes in your body temperature. In fact, daily body temperature increases right after ovulation, thus minimizing the normal decline in body temperature that occurs with sleep.[6]

- **Lower production of the natural sleep hormone melatonin** during the luteal phase, the second half of the menstrual cycle after ovulation,[7] which makes it harder to stay asleep at night and leaves you feeling sleepy the next day.

- **Pregnancy and child rearing** both take heavy tolls on a woman's sleep. One study revealed that women lose hundreds of hours of sleep during the first year of a child's life.[8] (And when their teenagers start driving, I'm sure worrying makes them lose hundreds of hours of sleep again!)

The susceptibility to hormone-related sleep problems waxes and wanes throughout a woman's life; sleep problems first surface during pregnancy and flare up again at perimenopause and menopause.

Along with female-specific sex hormones, imbalances of other substances in the body that affect mood, inflammation, and insulin balance can also contribute to poor sleep in women. Examples of these substances include the amino acid tryptophan and the sleep hormone melatonin. Tryptophan is necessary for the formation of serotonin, the neurotransmitter that has a calming influence in the brain.[9] Melatonin helps to regulate sleep cycles and sets the brain's biological clock. When levels of any or all of these substances fluctuate, the result can be a miserable night's sleep.

Why Women Can't Sleep: The Menstrual Cycle

According to a poll by the National Sleep Foundation, about 70 percent of menstruating women say their sleep is disrupted during their periods by symptoms like breast tenderness, bloating, cramps, and headaches.[10] The menstrual cycle is divided into four phases:

- **Menstrual phase**—Between the onset of your period (day 1 of your cycle) and its end
- **Follicular phase**—From the end of your period until ovulation at about day 14
- **Early luteal phase**—The week after ovulation (days 15 to 21)
- **Late luteal phase**—The time until menstruation starts again (days 22 to 28 or so)

At the start of your menstrual phase (when your period begins), there's a decline in estrogen (and a slowing of your metabolism) and you

NATURAL SLEEP TIPS FOR PMS AND YOUR PERIOD

1. **Increase your intake of liquids** to help flush out excess sodium that causes water retention and bloating just before and during your period. This will help decrease any feelings of discomfort that make sleep difficult.

2. **Take extra calcium.** In a study commissioned by the manufacturer of Tums (an OTC antacid medication containing calcium carbonate), taking 1,200 milligrams (mg) calcium daily resulted in a 50 percent decrease in PMS symptoms. Bloating was reduced by 36 percent, food cravings by 54 percent, and psychological symptoms by 46 percent. In addition, calcium has sedating properties, which can improve sleep quality.[11]

3. **Take 400 mg magnesium.** Studies show that magnesium affects mood by boosting the level of serotonin, the calming neurotransmitter in the brain. When combined with calcium, magnesium is a good muscle relaxant.[12] Of course, being relaxed is important to falling asleep easily.

4. **Take 100 mg vitamin B$_6$,** which also helps you produce serotonin. But be careful: In some people, B$_6$ can have an energizing effect.

5. **Starting at 2:00 p.m., eliminate all caffeine.** Caffeine is a stimulant that can trigger anxiety, making it difficult to fall asleep.

6. **Exercise in the early morning sunlight.** Remember, *do not exercise within 4 hours of bedtime.* Exercising close to bedtime can key you up and make it more difficult to fall asleep. However, getting outside in the natural sunlight can increase your melatonin level in the evening. In addition, getting sunlight each day is vital to keeping your serum vitamin D level adequate. We now know that sufficient vitamin D is important for producing leptin (the "stop" hormone that tells you to quit eating). I will explain more about this in Chapter 6.

7. **Don't drink alcohol within 3 hours of bedtime.** PMS can cause your blood level of alcohol to get higher than at other times of the month. While drinking alcohol may make you feel sleepier, alcohol also keeps you out of the deep stages of sleep, which are important for feeling refreshed when you awaken.

get sleepy. We now know that the drop in estrogen leads to less REM sleep, which is when dreams usually occur. Also, having a heavy period can lead to anemia from the lower iron level, which is a possible cause of restless legs syndrome—that uncomfortable creepy, crawly feeling you may get in your legs when you lie down that forces you to keep moving your legs or walking around.[13]

During the follicular phase, in the first half of your menstrual cycle, the brain signals the pituitary gland to make follicle-stimulating hormone, which triggers a rise in estrogen. Thus, you no longer feel sleepy—on the contrary, you may feel overly stimulated and have insomnia. During the follicular phase, women tend to have more light or poor-quality sleep (Stage 2) and an increase in REM sleep, often at the end of the night, which may make it difficult to wake up in the morning. So, it's both hard to fall asleep and hard to wake up during this menstrual phase leading to ovulation.

During the early luteal phase, the week after ovulation, the hormone progesterone is on the rise again. This will increase sleepiness and body temperature. Your circadian rhythm (which is controlled by melatonin) is affected. You will feel sleepy and want to go to bed earlier, but you will also wake up earlier. Your metabolism speeds up during this phase, so you will feel hungrier and eat more. Sleep will be lighter or of poorer quality.

In the final phase that leads up to menstruation—the late luteal phase, which is when many women experience PMS—estrogen and progesterone levels begin to fall back to normal, increasing awakenings and decreasing the amount of deep, restorative sleep you get and crave the most.

PMS Throws Off Your Biological Clock

To add to the trouble, it is thought that PMS also affects your biological clock by throwing off the timing of sleep, just as jet lag does. Normally, melatonin is low during the day and higher at night. However, in women dealing with PMS, melatonin is thought to be higher during the day, making them feel sleepy at the wrong time.

While in the throes of PMS, some women say they feel fatigued no

LIGHT THERAPY, HORMONES, AND SLEEP

It is well documented that light entering the eyes influences the pituitary and pineal glands, which control the entire endocrine system, the system that produces substances affecting metabolism. At night, when it is dark, the brain generates less serotonin and more melatonin. But light therapy, using natural or artificial light, can cause physiological changes in the human body.

With light therapy, a particular kind of light called broad-spectrum light that is emitted by a "light box" is used to simulate the effect of a few extra hours of sunlight each day. People exposed to it subsequently produce serotonin.

Because of this boost in serotonin, light therapy can sometimes ease depression, which in many cases produces sleep disorders (sleeping too much or not being able to stay asleep). Light therapy is often used to relieve the symptoms associated with seasonal affective disorder (SAD), a psychological problem that occurs during times of the year with less daytime light. I talk more about SAD in Chapter 6.

In light-therapy studies, women with PMS reported less depression, less moodiness, better sleep, and better concentration after treatment.[14] Researchers have shown that the drop in serotonin production just before ovulation correlates with the onset of PMS symptoms.[15] The serotonin level then rebounds with the onset of menstruation, which is when PMS symptoms decrease. Some findings show that PMS symptoms occur more often in women with low base levels of serotonin.[16, 17] When the level of serotonin drops before ovulation, it gets low enough for serious symptoms to appear. By using light therapy, these women can keep their serotonin and melatonin levels high enough to prevent their PMS symptoms from appearing.

matter how long they stay in bed. In addition, a study showed that women who experienced PMS rated their alertness as significantly lower during both menstrual phases studied (the follicular phase and the late luteal, premenstrual phase).[18] *It may be that the lower level of alertness is due to a tendency toward poorer sleep in women with PMS.* Studies show that women have more awakenings, sleep disturbances, and vivid dreams with PMS than they do during the rest of the month.

PMS tends to occur more often in women from ages 26 to 42 who have had at least one child and have a family history of depression and/or a past medical history of postpartum depression or a mood disorder.[19]

Women with severe PMS (also called premenstrual dysphoric disorder, or PMDD) report even more sleep-related complaints, including having trouble falling and staying asleep, fatigue, sluggishness, and difficulty concentrating. In fact, sleep disturbance—either being sleepy all the time or having trouble getting to sleep or staying asleep—is one of the defining criteria for a diagnosis of PMDD.

Pregnancy and Postpartum Sleep (Or Lack of It)

Among women of childbearing age (approximately ages 15 through 44), pregnant women are among the *least likely* to enjoy a good night's sleep. Now, I am not suggesting at all that you should pursue better sleep during pregnancy to lose weight. As your obstetrician will tell you, you need to eat well-balanced meals and enough calories to maintain a healthy pregnancy. However, I do know that better sleep will help you make the right nutritional choices. In fact, as we've discussed, people who sleep fewer than 5.5 hours at night crave more carbs and snacks—mostly at nighttime.

! SLEEP
! ALERT

A study from the University of California at San Francisco revealed that women who got fewer than 6 hours of sleep per night had longer labors and increased risk of Caesarean sections—all the more reason to **focus on getting good sleep** so you stay rested throughout your pregnancy and are fully prepared for the grand event.[20]

The greatest sleep variations during pregnancy usually occur during the first and third trimesters. Not only does the surge of sleep-inducing progesterone make you feel sleepy all day long and cause imbalance among all your hormones, but also the growing fetus applies pressure on the bladder, making nighttime visits to the bathroom more common.

Also, many pregnant women have a digestive disorder called gastro-esophageal reflux disease (GERD), in which stomach acid gets into the esophagus. The problem, often referred to as heartburn, is worsened by the pressure the growing fetus puts on the mother's internal organs. One study found that 30 to 50 percent of pregnant women experience GERD almost constantly during pregnancy.[21] Normally, a muscle called a sphincter that lies between the esophagus and the stomach prevents stomach acid from backing up into the esophagus. In those with GERD, this sphincter does not work properly. The stomach acid backs up—"refluxes"—into the esophagus, causing irritation and inflammation. If the acid that gets into the esophagus makes it to the trachea and then to the lungs, inflammation and a certain type of pneumonia can result. Since this reflux generally occurs at night when you are lying down, it further disrupts your already disrupted sleep.

Let's review each trimester to see how pregnancy affects your sleep.

1st Trimester

- You may experience excessive sleepiness because of the increased secretion of progesterone.
- After the first 6 to 8 weeks, you may have insomnia—specifically, more awakenings throughout the night (often to go to the bathroom).
- Heartburn may interrupt good sleep.
- You may have difficulty sleeping because of nausea, breast tenderness, and backache.

2nd Trimester

- Sleep usually improves during this time. Your body seems to be getting used to the changed hormone levels.
- Some women experience fetal movement, which may wake them up at night (babies have their own schedules!).
- Heartburn may continue to disrupt sleep.
- Deep-sleep time begins to shorten, and some women experience restless legs.

3rd Trimester

- As your belly gets bigger, breathing becomes more difficult and GERD and other physical discomforts worsen.
- Hormonal changes that prepare you to deliver the baby result in even more sleep disturbances, including nightmares in some women.
- Sciatic nerve pain caused by pressure from the enlarged uterus may cause lower-back and/or leg pain that disrupt sleep.
- Anxiety about becoming a mother may cause insomnia.

Postpartum Sleeplessness

The 6 to 8 weeks following childbirth is a sleepless time for most moms—and a busy time for sleep doctors, as women call them seeking remedies for themselves and their newborns. A revealing study showed that at 1 year postpartum, new moms who slept less than 5 hours during a 24-hour period were more likely to be carrying extra weight.[22] Getting 1 to 2 more hours of sleep each day is just as important as diet and exercise in helping you to lose that baby fat. While it may be tough managing 7 to 8 hours of sleep with a new baby, your weight depends upon getting adequate sleep every night.

Dana, 38, called my clinic 6 weeks after delivering her second baby. She said that her first son, Eric, slept well and had been sleeping about 10 hours a night by 6 weeks (don't worry, he was also napping during the day to get his required 18-plus hours). But her newborn, Justin, had colic. Whenever Justin wasn't being held by Dana or her husband, he cried nonstop.

Since Dana was breastfeeding, she was on duty all alone each night. By 6 weeks, she had seriously disrupted sleep. She said that when she fed the baby, she would treat herself to a snack. As a result, she had lost only 3 pounds since she was released from the hospital.

NATURAL SLEEP TIPS
FOR POSTPARTUM MOMS

- Learn techniques that will help you relax. Increased relaxation will improve both your bonding with your newborn and your sleep.
- Take naps when you can.
- Eat your largest meal during the day rather than at night.
- Eat foods high in tryptophan (see page 175).
- Ask others to help out; you can't do everything on your own.
- Avoid caffeine after 2:00 p.m. so you can feel drowsy when it's time to go to bed.
- Get outside in the morning sunlight to help set your biological clock.

NATURAL SLEEP TIPS FOR PREGNANCY

Use these tips to sleep longer and make better nutritional choices at meal and snack times during pregnancy.

1st Trimester

- Schedule and prioritize sleep. Add daytime naps. You will need them.
- Drink plenty of fluids throughout the day, but cut back on the amount before bedtime. This can help avoid nighttime urination.
- Eat bland snacks to avoid having nausea disturb your naps or nighttime sleep.
- Sleep on your left side, because this can improve the flow of nutrient-rich blood to the fetus.
- Put a night-light in the bathroom so you won't need to turn on a light to use the bathroom. The dim night-light will be less arousing and help you return to sleep more quickly. But make sure the night-light provides enough light that you can see what you are doing.

2nd Trimester

- Avoid eating spicy, acidic, or fried foods to keep stomach acid at bay. Sleep with your head elevated on two pillows. Eat frequent, small meals to reduce heartburn or GERD.
- Enjoy your 2nd trimester sleep! Get as close to 8 hours a night as possible.
- Take pressure off your lower back. Lie on your side with your legs bent at the knees and hips. Place pillows between your knees, under your abdomen, and behind your back.
- Talk to a therapist or counselor if nightmares or disturbing dreams are causing you distress.

3rd Trimester

- Sleep on your left side.
- Check out pregnancy pillows and find one that works for you.
- If you start snoring, have your blood pressure and urine protein level checked.
- If you develop leg restlessness, talk to your ob/gyn about a possible iron deficiency. If you can't sleep at night, get up and read a book, write in a journal, or take a warm bath.
- Avoid carbonated drinks if you have leg cramps. If you do get a cramp in your leg, straighten it and flex your foot upward for relief.

Once a sweet, effervescent person, Dana was now irritable, even angry at times. Unable to fall asleep, she walked the house at night listening for Justin's cries. She felt like she could fall asleep at any time, even when driving.

Before Justin's birth, Dana had been too busy tending to her first-born, Eric, to get all the sleep she really needed. So, she had accumulated a huge sleep debt before Justin was born, and because of his colic and inability to sleep, her sleep debt only worsened in the weeks after delivery. She found herself blaming her newborn and began having difficulty bonding with him. When she called me, she asked for a few strategies to help Justin sleep, but I knew when she told me about her inability to sleep that I would be working on both of them.

Here are the tips I gave her in this tough situation.

1. Since Dana wanted to breastfeed, I asked if she'd considered using a breast pump. She could pump her breast milk during the day and let her husband feed the baby with a bottle at night. This would allow Dana to get some sleep when she needed rest the most.

2. To that end, we created an "on call" schedule. In much the same way a doctor is on call, I explained to her, her husband could be tasked with feeding Justin at certain times during the day or night so Dana could rest.

3. I suggested that she not worry about doing other household chores and instead sleep whenever her baby did. Laundry can always be done later, I told her, but if she napped when Justin napped, she would feel better.

4. Exercising was another suggestion I gave her. I recommended that she walk in the early morning sunlight with Justin in a stroller. This would allow Dana to get some exercise and socialize with other moms. It also would help the baby sleep better,

but, more important, exercising in the sunlight would have a beneficial effect on her depression.

5. I gave Dana some tips on foods to keep on hand that might calm her at night and increase her drowsiness, such as unsalted almonds, crackers with cheese, and fat-free milk (her mom had given her warm milk at night as a child, and it still comforted her). If she substituted these healthier snacks instead of indulging her usual cookie cravings, she might see faster weight loss.

A National Sleep Foundation poll showed that 55 percent of postpartum women reported getting a good night's sleep only a few nights a month or less and 84 percent reported symptoms of insomnia.[23] When asked what awakened them most during the night, 90 percent of postpartum women said "giving care to a child." This sleep deprivation can have serious consequences, as evidenced by the 20 percent of postpartum women who said they had driven drowsy with children in the car and the 19 percent of women like Dana who said they experienced postpartum blues or depression. During the postpartum period, a woman's body is going through incredible hormonal changes. Throughout pregnancy, estrogen and progesterone levels are elevated; however, these levels return to normal in the first 24 hours after delivery.[24]

One of the sleep problems that occur during the postpartum period is nighttime awakening. When a new mother gets up at night and turns on an ordinary light to take care of her baby, her pineal gland may stop making melatonin.[25] Light signals the brain to wake up.

When the new mom goes back to bed, she can have trouble falling asleep because her brain thinks it is morning. If this happens several times a night, as it normally does, the woman is apt to produce little melatonin. Or, if the pattern occurs for many consecutive nights (as happened with Dana), there can be disruption of the new mom's circadian rhythms, which can even lead to depression.

SLEEP 101

HOW TO HAVE A GREAT AFTERNOON NAP

- Find a quiet place where noise, phones, and people will not interrupt you.
- Start your nap before 3:00 p.m.; otherwise, you might have trouble sleeping at night. Make sure you have taken a couple of hours after lunch to digest your meal before you lie down for your nap.
- Make sure the room is a comfortable temperature, between 68°F and 72°F. Have a light blanket nearby if necessary.
- Make sure the room is somewhat dim and not in direct sunlight.
- Take off your shoes and turn off your phone and any other electronics. Use an eyeshade or earplugs if necessary.
- Set an alarm for 30 minutes, just enough time for you to rest without entering a deep-sleep phase.

Interestingly, one team of scientists from Ohio-based John Carroll University found that new mothers who want to reduce their chances of postpartum blues need to block out the *blue rays of light* that cause melatonin suppression. The scientists have developed special lightbulbs for a baby's nursery as well as special glasses that they say can help new mothers avoid sleep deprivation and perhaps depression.[26] It is thought that blue light's wavelength (460–480 nanometers) affects certain receptors in the eye that inhibit the production of melatonin.

Is Infertility Linked to Sleep Deprivation?

Have you ever considered that infertility might be linked to poor sleep? The word "infertility" can quickly generate a response, especially among the 10 percent (more than 6 million) of women of childbearing age struggling with conception. Yet a 2008 report reveals that not getting enough sleep can impact your ability to conceive.[27] Here's why.

- Sleep has a powerful influence on the body's hormonal system, which controls a woman's menstrual cycle and regulates ovulation.
- Too little sleep leads to a low level of leptin. Remember leptin? It is the appetite hormone that stops your hunger. Preliminary research shows that having a low level of leptin may signal the brain to shut down nonessential functions like ovulation. In turn, many women with ovulation problems have difficulty getting pregnant.
- Insomniacs have significantly higher levels of the stress hormones cortisol and adrenocorticotropin,[28] both of which can suppress fertility.

The take-home message is clear: You could be doing everything right when it comes to preparing your body to conceive and bring a healthy baby to term. But there may be a missing link, even with all the focus on external factors like your environment and what you eat. The time has come to add another element to this formula: *sleep.*

If you have insomnia, ask your fertility specialist about the fertility medication you are taking to see if it could be causing your sleep problem. Sometimes medications such as clomiphene (Clomid, Serophene) cause hot flashes that work against getting a good night's sleep.

Midlife Insomnia and Weight Gain

A great many of the women who come to me with sleep issues are perimenopausal. These women, usually in their early to midforties, often complain of an inability to sleep or restlessness that keeps them from relaxing so they can sleep. In fact, more than half (59 percent) of women in this life stage say they experience symptoms of insomnia at least a few nights each week.[29] I find that there is a high correlation between poor sleep and weight gain (usually as belly fat) in women at midlife. The problem with an expanding waistline at this life stage is that it increases your risks of heart disease, diabetes, and certain types of cancers.[30]

SLEEP 101

TRY THE 20-MINUTE NAP-A-LATTE

Need to get through a long day but don't want to overdo it on the caffeine? I often recommend the **Nap-a-Latte** to patients. You can take a Nap-a-Latte anytime before 2:00 p.m. (any later and it might keep you from sleeping that night). Here's what you do.

1. Drink 1 cup of cool coffee or black tea quickly (make sure you get about 90 to 100 mg of caffeine).
2. Lie down and take a 20-minute nap.

When you wake up, the caffeine should be kicking in, and you will have gotten some rest while waiting. This little double shot of rest and caffeine should take you through the remainder of the afternoon.

Granted, the Nap-a-Latte may not be an option at work unless you have an office door you can close. But you can take a nap during a lunch break by sleeping in your car if you can set your cell phone or wristwatch alarm to wake you up after 20 minutes. Remember, always be safe when napping in a car.

Sleep disturbances, from hot flashes to night sweats, occur in 39 to 47 percent of women during perimenopause (the time before menopause) and in 35 to 60 percent of postmenopausal women.[31] Some women report that hot flashes occur for several months; for others, these disruptions last for several years if they start at the beginning of perimenopause. Adding to many women's stress at this life stage is juggling responsibilities for careers, kids, and aging parents. Others are dealing with personal health problems—all of which can add to anxiety and result in feelings of overload, poor sleep, and obesity.

With aging, the prevalence of insomnia increases as sleep time decreases, even though the time spent in bed may increase. As millions of women report at midlife, it takes longer to fall asleep and is harder to stay asleep. The result is daytime sleepiness, irritability, difficulty concentrating, and poor performance.

In perimenopause, the declining level of the hormone estradiol may increase the chance of poor sleep (estradiol acts like a growth hormone for the tissues of reproductive organs). In a study published in the journal *Obstetrics and Gynecology*, researchers followed 436 women ages 35 to 49 over a 2-year period.[32] About 17 percent of the women reported having poor sleep throughout the entire study period. While researchers blamed anxiety, depression, and caffeine consumption as factors that disturbed the women's sleep, they also identified low estradiol levels and hot flashes in women ages 45 to 49 as contributing to the sleepless nights. Interestingly, these women were still having regular periods and had not yet entered perimenopause. The researchers concluded that the decline in estradiol that occurs with ovarian aging might be associated with poor sleep. This poor sleep results in daytime fatigue and irritability, weight gain, and sometimes depression.

Menopause, Night Sweats, and No Sleep

When Marnie, age 50, came to my clinic, she had been plagued for months by hot flashes that woke her up several times each night. She not only was sick of the resulting daytime fatigue and irritability, but also felt old and fat because her waistline had expanded 3½ inches in less than a year. Initially, she came to me for some strategies to help her stay asleep and wake up feeling refreshed. But along with improving her sleep, the changes I recommended resulted in her dropping 9 pounds in 1 month *without changing her diet.* She felt rested and more energetic, and the extra bonus of weight loss helped her to feel good about herself again. Here are the sleep tips I gave her to boost her sleep at midlife.

- **Keep the bedroom temperature between 68°F and 72°F, if possible.** Marnie was keeping her bedroom at 65°F, but hot flashes stem from an internal, physiological process and have little to do with a room's temperature. In fact, the cooler temperature of

Marnie's bedroom actually worsened how she felt at night. For example, she would sweat to cool her body during a hot flash. But once the cold air hit the sweat, the water cooled on her skin, creating the same effect as getting out of a swimming pool on a cold day. Brrr.

- **Add soy products to your diet.** The isoflavones in soy products have an estrogen-like effect on the body. Some findings show that women who eat soy products report fewer hot flashes than women who do not eat soy do.[33] Fewer hot flashes may increase sound sleep.

In less than 2 weeks, Marnie began to notice a difference in her temperature fluctuations and nighttime awakenings. With improved sleep, she began to feel energetic again and was able to exercise more and be more physically active.

Menopause occurs at an average age of 51, though it's earlier in some women and later in others. Perimenopause is an ongoing process of physical change that usually starts about 10 years before your periods end entirely.

At menopause, your body curtails its production of both estrogen and progesterone, yet estrogen never disappears from your system completely; your ovaries, adrenal glands, and fatty tissues continue to manufacture small amounts of other hormones that your body converts into forms of estrogen.

The most bothersome parts of menopause are the uncomfortable symptoms (hot flashes, night sweats, and vaginal dryness, among many others), which can vary greatly among women. During the period leading into and after menopause, a reported 75 percent of women have hot flashes, and about 22 percent of them have problems sleeping at least a few nights a week because of the hot flashes and night sweats.[34] Severe hot flashes can be linked to chronic insomnia at this life stage.[35, 36]

Weight gain after menopause can also cause sleep loss. The fat that many women gain in their necks can be significant enough to hinder breathing and in some cases can contribute to the development of sleep apnea.[37]

Sleep disturbances and weight problems in midlife may also be related to the aging process or problems such as depression and thyroid dysfunction. It's important not to assume that poor sleep or even a diagnosable sleep disorder is just another menopause symptom.[38] Sleep problems—no matter how insignificant they seem—are serious and warrant discussion with your health care provider.

Finding Your Optimal Sleep Temperature

The key to a good night's sleep for most women is often as easy as regulating the thermostat. While this is particularly important for women during perimenopause, all women can benefit from this important sleep strategy. A growing area of research is the effect of external temperature on sleep. Much of this research has shown that the optimal temperature for sleep is between 65°F and 75°F.[39] You know that a drop in core body temperature triggers sleepiness, and external temperatures in this range help to induce it. In fact, temperatures that are too far out of this range can have the opposite effect and cause restlessness.[40]

Studies have shown that before bed, a normal sleeper has a lower body temperature than an insomniac; this higher temperature in an insomniac causes him or her difficulty in falling asleep as the body struggles to reset its thermostat.[41] When a normal sleeper's core temperature drops, blood vessels dilate to radiate the extra heat, so the temperature of the hands and feet increases.[42] People who experience difficulty sleeping have been shown to benefit from having a cool bedroom and a hot-water bottle by their feet to quickly dilate the blood vessels, thereby helping to lower the core temperature.

Natural Sleep Tips for Menopause and Beyond

- Dress in lightweight sleepwear. Try sleepwear made out of a moisture-wicking fabric, a microdenier material similar to silk that pulls perspiration away from your body.
- Avoid heavy blankets. Believe it or not, wool works quite nicely year-round.
- Consider using a room fan or air conditioning to cool the air and increase its circulation, but do not set your thermostat below 65°F (see the "Sleep Tip" on page 76). A colder temperature will actually disrupt your sleep, not help you sleep more soundly.
- Reduce stress to stay cool and calm.
- Try relaxation techniques, including massage and exercise.
- Talk to a behavioral health professional if you are depressed, anxious, or having emotional issues.

Postmenopausal Sleep Disorders

Did you know that women who are postmenopausal have the highest BMIs of all adults, with 36 percent of them being overweight and another 30 percent obese?[43] Is it any wonder that studies show that up to 61 percent of healthy women over the age of 60 report sleep disturbance and poor sleep quality?[44] I treat many postmenopausal women—not so much for hormone-related issues, but rather for more serious sleep disorders such as sleep apnea, restless legs syndrome, and insomnia.

During aging and postmenopausally, sleep becomes more shallow or

SLEEP 101

There are many different theories about the optimal bedroom temperature for sleep. I have always recommended trying to keep the bedroom between 68°F and 72°F. This was based on a study that concluded that sleep was negatively affected when the room temperature was either below 65°F or above 75°F.

Although those temperatures are good benchmarks, there does not seem to be a right temperature for optimal sleep for everyone. Furthermore, the ideal temperature changes throughout the night. For most people, core body temperature tends to decrease at about 11:00 p.m., hit its lowest temperature at about 4:00 a.m., and then slowly rise to the waking temperature. This pattern can change if you have extensive exposure to light, exercise in the late evening, or are a shift worker, or do not keep a regular sleep schedule.[45]

Generally speaking, a cooler room is usually better. However, keeping to a consistent temperature that is comfortable for both you and your bed partner is an important factor in experiencing good-quality sleep.

There is also a second microclimate to consider—under your covers. Remember, your body will adapt to its surrounding temperature until uncomfortable, at which time it will either: wake you from deep sleep if cold, to move and create friction, or wake you from deep sleep if warm, to remove covers and ventilate.

So I often counsel women to make sure their microclimate is just right, usually low to mid 80s.

light and is more easily interrupted.[46] It has also been shown that 61 percent of postmenopausal women have symptoms of insomnia at least a few nights each week, with 22 percent of postmenopausal women saying they have a difficult time sleeping due to hot flashes or night sweats. In fact, findings show that 41 percent of postmenopausal women say they resort to a prescription or OTC sleep aid at least a few nights per week.[47]

Postmenopausal women have the highest incidence of sleep apnea.[48] While it used to be thought that it was their higher BMIs and larger necks that put these women at risk for the disorder, research shows that perimenopausal and postmenopausal women have functional, rather than anatomic, differences in their upper airways. This altered functioning of the airway as you age may cause apnea.[49] Weight loss is recommended to reduce the risk of sleep apnea,[50] and better sleep can help you to lose weight once and for all.

Part II

Sleep Yourself THINNER: THE PLAN

5

Diagnose Your Sleep Deficits

We all want to wake up refreshed so we can go about our day with energy, a clear mind, and a positive outlook. But before you can make any changes to fix your sleep problems, you need to find out what is really disturbing your sleep.

Keeping a *Sleep Diary* has helped many of my patients keep track of their sleep and see how their lifestyle habits and behavior affect how well they sleep. In this brief chapter, I will tell you how to review your current sleep situation by keeping a Sleep Diary for 2 weeks. By accounting for lifestyle factors such as how much you exercised, how much caffeine you consumed, and what you ate and then comparing these to your sleep patterns, you can see which parameters impact your sleep (or lack of it!).

Here's how the Sleep Diary works: Using the Sleep Diary forms pages at the end of this chapter, I'd like you to keep track of your lifestyle habits, including your diet and exercise regimen, every day for at least 2 weeks. I also want you to note the time you go to bed and the time you wake up. Write down how long you think it took you to fall asleep, how many times you awakened during the night, and how you felt when you woke up in the morning. Record the total number of hours you slept in addition to describing what kinds of sleep disturbances you had. You should also note what you were doing 1 hour before going to bed, any medication you took that day, what you ate and drank within 2 to 3 hours of going bed, when you exercised, and how much caffeine you consumed.

After keeping a Sleep Diary for at least 2 weeks, review the entries to get a better idea of your sleep hygiene, your sleep quality, and what you need to do to improve your nighttime slumber. Do you notice any sleep "stumbling blocks"? Once you identify specific barriers to good sleep, you can then use strategies to prepare your mind, body, and bedroom for a delicious night's sleep. We call these strategies *sleep hygiene,* which refers to the habits, environmental factors, and even rituals that can help you to get sound sleep. Do you drink too much caffeine throughout the day? Do you exercise right before bedtime and find yourself all keyed up and unable to relax? Maybe you lack a regular sleep regimen; you should allow yourself time for sleep hygiene before bed to set the tone for sleep. Or perhaps you leave the TV on in your bedroom and it keeps you from falling asleep once you start feeling drowsy.

Observing careful sleep hygiene habits each night is critical for many women, but particularly so for women who are very *sensitive sleepers* and require the perfect bed and sleep environment to get good-quality sleep. Sleep hygiene habits are also important for women who have a hard time calming their minds at night and need to slowly ease into their bedtime routines.

These things will not only help you avoid behaviors that lead to weight gain, but also improve your overall quality of life immeasurably. I truly believe that the key to great sleep is practicing good sleep hygiene so that you can fall asleep quickly—and predictably—on most nights. When you look at your bedroom as your personal sleep sanctuary, you will find that a good night's sleep becomes much easier to attain.

Rita, 35, a busy mom of two and elementary school teacher, cannot fall asleep unless her bedtime prerequisites are perfect by her lofty standards. This includes making sure her nightclothes, the sheets and pillows, the room temperature, and more are all exactly the way she likes them to be. If one of her bedtime requirements is off, Rita feels anxious and hyperalert, which only makes it more difficult for her to relax and fall asleep. Because she realizes that she's a supersensitive sleeper, Rita starts her nightly routine about an hour before bedtime with the following actions.

- Pulling back the comforter and top sheet on her bed and fluffing and arranging her two pillows to suit her taste
- Setting the thermostat at 68°F, because she likes her bedroom cool and dry
- Turning off all the lights in the bedroom and hallway, pulling down the blackout shades in the bedroom, and turning on the white noise sound machine
- Setting her earplugs and sleep mask on her pillow to put on when she gets in bed
- Doing 10 minutes of yoga postures and stretching that improve breathing and flexibility
- Washing her face to remove her makeup, applying moisturizer, and then, in dim light, massaging her neck, shoulders, and forehead to ease muscle tension and increase relaxation
- Taking a warm bath only by the light of several large scented candles flickering near the tub
- Putting on her ultrasoft nightclothes and finally being ready for good sleep

SLEEP **QUIZ**

THINGS THAT GO BUMP IN THE NIGHT: TAKE THE SLEEP DISRUPTION QUIZ

Do you know what disrupts your sleep each night? Take the **Sleep Disruption Quiz** to get a better idea of problems that can compromise the quantity and quality of your sleep. Below are descriptions of common sleep disruptions. Check all of the ones that keep you from getting the rest you need. Give yourself 1 point if the problem describes you and 0 if it does not. Add up your score to determine how bad (or good) your sleep quality might be.

1. Frequent arousals during a night's sleep for unknown reasons
2. Sudden awakening in the middle of the night to answer a child's cries and not being able to get back to sleep
3. Difficulty falling asleep because your bed partner is snoring
4. A new reduction in total sleep time (for example, from 7 hours to 6)
5. Long awakenings (10 minutes or longer) during the night
6. Awakening with night sweats or hot flashes
7. Awakening in the morning feeling exhausted and foggy
8. Feeling anxious and fearful about sleep
9. Glancing at the clock on the nightstand throughout the night
10. Frequent tossing and turning because of an old, lumpy, or too thin mattress
11. Discomfort because of scratchy, rough sheets
12. Getting less than 6 hours of sleep on most nights
13. Frequent awakenings caused by your own nasal allergies and snoring
14. Difficulty sleeping because of one or more pets in your bed
15. Discomfort because the bedroom is too cold, too warm, too humid, or too dry
16. Difficulty sleeping while traveling
17. Being mentally alert during the night as you ruminate about problems and fears or nothing at all

18. Being unable to sleep because of noises either inside the house or outside

19. Sleep problems caused by drinking caffeinated or alcoholic beverages too close to bedtime

Now total up your score:

14 to 19: Talk to your doctor. You may have a sleep disorder (page 33) that needs medical attention. You can take advantage of the natural sleep solutions in this book, too.

6 to 13: You will benefit from the natural sleep solutions that follow. You'll learn to de-stress, calm hormone havoc, eat to boost calming neurotransmitters, and exercise outdoors to benefit from sunlight. If you have symptoms of a sleep disorder or are concerned about pain, snoring, or anxiety, see your doctor for a medical assessment.

0 to 5: Your sleep problems are not too bad! Your sleep probably reflects healthy choices you have made during adulthood. Keep up your healthy lifestyle habits and use some of my natural sleep solutions to remedy any problems you may have with your sleep hygiene.

Are you a highly sensitive sleeper like Rita who needs time to unwind and relax before bed? Did your sleep diary reveal that you need to cut out caffeine or exercise earlier in the day or turn off the TV before the nightly news? In the next chapter, I want to focus on the *Sleep Doctor's 5 Simple Rules* and how these very specific rules work to almost guarantee you a better night's sleep and subsequent weight loss.

No matter what stumbling blocks you identify, you will find excellent answers in this part of *The Sleep Doctor's Diet Plan.*

Your Sleep Diary

WEEK 1

	MON	TUES	WED	THURS	FRI	SAT	SUN
DATE →							
I went to bed at: (give clock time)	__:__ m	__:__ m	__:__ m	__:__ m	__:__ m	__:__ m	__:__ m
I fell asleep at: (guess clock time)	__:__ m	__:__ m	__:__ m	__:__ m	__:__ m	__:__ m	__:__ m
I woke up for the day at: (give clock time)	__:__ m	__:__ m	__:__ m	__:__ m	__:__ m	__:__ m	__:__ m
How many times did you wake up last night?							
How many naps did you take yesterday? (give number)							
How long did your naps last? (give total number of minutes)							
Sleep **Quality**: 1. Very poor 2. Poor 3. OK 4. Good 5. Very good							
Sleep **Quantity**: 1. Very inadequate 2. Inadequate 3. About right 4. Too much							
I woke up **feeling refreshed.** 1. Not at all 2. Somewhat 3. A little 4. Yes 5. Very							
How many alcoholic beverages did you have last night?							
How many alcoholic beverages did you have 3 hours before bed?							

	MON	TUES	WED	THURS	FRI	SAT	SUN
DATE →							
How many caffein-ated beverages did you drink yesterday?							
How many caffeinated beverages did you have after 2 p.m.?							
How many minutes of direct sunlight did you get yesterday?							
Did you exercise yesterday? If yes, was it less than 4 hours before bed?							
Did you go to bed within 30 min of your predicted sleep need?							
Did you wake up before your alarm today? 1. Yes 2. No							

Notes_____

_____

_____

_____

_____

_____

_____

WEEK 2

	MON	TUES	WED	THURS	FRI	SAT	SUN
DATE →							
I went to bed at: (give clock time)	__:__ _m	__:__ _m	__:__ _m	__:__ _m	__:__ _m	__:__ _m	__:__ _m
I fell asleep at: (guess clock time)	__:__ _m	__:__ _m	__:__ _m	__:__ _m	__:__ _m	__:__ _m	__:__ _m
I woke up for the day at: (give clock time)	__:__ _m	__:__ _m	__:__ _m	__:__ _m	__:__ _m	__:__ _m	__:__ _m
How many times did you wake up last night?							
How many naps did you take yesterday? (give number)							
How long did your naps last? (give total number of minutes)							
Sleep **Quality**: 1. Very poor 2. Poor 3. OK 4. Good 5. Very good							
Sleep **Quantity**: 1. Very inadequate 2. Inadequate 3. About right 4. Too much							
I woke up **feeling refreshed.** 1. Not at all 2. Somewhat 3. A little 4. Yes 5. Very							
How many alcoholic beverages did you have last night?							
How many alcoholic beverages did you have 3 hours before bed?							
How many caffein-ated beverages did you drink yesterday?							

	MON	TUES	WED	THURS	FRI	SAT	SUN
DATE →							
How many caffeinated beverages did you have after 2 p.m.?							
How many minutes of direct sunlight did you get yesterday?							
Did you exercise yesterday? If yes, was it less than 4 hours before bed?							
Did you go to bed within 30 min of your predicted sleep need?							
Did you wake up before your alarm today? 1. Yes 2. No							

Notes_____

_____

_____

_____

_____

_____

_____

_____

_____

_____

_____

_____

_____

_____

WEEK 3

	MON	TUES	WED	THURS	FRI	SAT	SUN
DATE →							
I went to bed at: (give clock time)	__:___m	__:___m	__:___m	__:___m	__:___m	__:___m	__:___m
I fell asleep at: (guess clock time)	__:___m	__:___m	__:___m	__:___m	__:___m	__:___m	__:___m
I woke up for the day at: (give clock time)	__:___m	__:___m	__:___m	__:___m	__:___m	__:___m	__:___m
How many times did you wake up last night?							
How many naps did you take yesterday? (give number)							
How long did your naps last? (give total number of minutes)							
Sleep **Quality**: 1. Very poor 2. Poor 3. OK 4. Good 5. Very good							
Sleep **Quantity**: 1. Very inadequate 2. Inadequate 3. About right 4. Too much							
I woke up **feeling refreshed**. 1. Not at all 2. Somewhat 3. A little 4. Yes 5. Very							
How many alcoholic beverages did you have last night?							
How many alcoholic beverages did you have 3 hours before bed?							
How many caffeinated beverages did you drink yesterday?							

	MON	TUES	WED	THURS	FRI	SAT	SUN
DATE →							
How many caffeinated beverages did you have after 2 p.m.?							
How many minutes of direct sunlight did you get yesterday?							
Did you exercise yesterday? If yes, was it less than 4 hours before bed?							
Did you go to bed within 30 min of your predicted sleep need?							
Did you wake up before your alarm today? 1. Yes 2. No							

Notes
_____
_____
_____
_____
_____
_____
_____
_____
_____
_____
_____
_____
_____
_____
_____

WEEK 4

	MON	TUES	WED	THURS	FRI	SAT	SUN
DATE →							
I went to bed at: (give clock time)	__:___m	__:___m	__:___m	__:___m	__:___m	__:___m	__:___m
I fell asleep at: (guess clock time)	__:___m	__:___m	__:___m	__:___m	__:___m	__:___m	__:___m
I woke up for the day at: (give clock time)	__:___m	__:___m	__:___m	__:___m	__:___m	__:___m	__:___m
How many times did you wake up last night?							
How many naps did you take yesterday? (give number)							
How long did your naps last? (give total number of minutes)							
Sleep **Quality**: 1. Very poor 2. Poor 3. OK 4. Good 5. Very good							
Sleep **Quantity**: 1. Very inadequate 2. Inadequate 3. About right 4. Too much							
I woke up **feeling refreshed.** 1. Not at all 2. Somewhat 3. A little 4. Yes 5. Very							
How many alcoholic beverages did you have last night?							
How many alcoholic beverages did you have 3 hours before bed?							
How many caffeinated beverages did you drink yesterday?							

	MON	TUES	WED	THURS	FRI	SAT	SUN
DATE ➔							
How many caffeinated beverages did you have after 2 p.m.?							
How many minutes of direct sunlight did you get yesterday?							
Did you exercise yesterday? If yes, was it less than 4 hours before bed?							
Did you go to bed within 30 min of your predicted sleep need?							
Did you wake up before your alarm today? 1. Yes 2. No							

Notes_____

_____

_____

_____

_____

_____

_____

_____

_____

_____

_____

_____

_____

_____

_____

WEEK 5

	MON	TUES	WED	THURS	FRI	SAT	SUN
DATE ➔							
I went to bed at: (give clock time)	__:___m	__:___m	__:___m	__:___m	__:___m	__:___m	__:___m
I fell asleep at: (guess clock time)	__:___m	__:___m	__:___m	__:___m	__:___m	__:___m	__:___m
I woke up for the day at: (give clock time)	__:___m	__:___m	__:___m	__:___m	__:___m	__:___m	__:___m
How many times did you wake up last night?							
How many naps did you take yesterday? (give number)							
How long did your naps last? (give total number of minutes)							
Sleep **Quality**: 1. Very poor 2. Poor 3. OK 4. Good 5. Very good							
Sleep **Quantity**: 1. Very inadequate 2. Inadequate 3. About right 4. Too much							
I woke up **feeling refreshed.** 1. Not at all 2. Somewhat 3. A little 4. Yes 5. Very							
How many alcoholic beverages did you have last night?							
How many alcoholic beverages did you have 3 hours before bed?							
How many caffeinated beverages did you drink yesterday?							

	MON	TUES	WED	THURS	FRI	SAT	SUN
DATE ➔							
How many caffeinated beverages did you have after 2 p.m.?							
How many minutes of direct sunlight did you get yesterday?							
Did you exercise yesterday? If yes, was it less than 4 hours before bed?							
Did you go to bed within 30 min of your predicted sleep need?							
Did you wake up before your alarm today? 1. Yes 2. No							

Notes_____

_____

_____

_____

_____

_____

_____

_____

_____

_____

_____

_____

_____

_____

_____

6

The 5 Simple Rules
for Better Sleep

Sleep hygiene is a collection of behaviors that promote better sleep. By using good sleep hygiene regularly, you can see how what you do during the daytime hours affects the quality of your sleep at night. Traditionally, sleep hygiene researchers focused on recommending that people avoid three substances—alcohol, nicotine, and caffeine—and keep a regular bedtime. However, today sleep scientists know that a host of other behaviors also affect sleep. I base the *Sleep Doctor's 5 Simple Rules* on the principles of good sleep hygiene. They are as easy as 1, 2, 3, 4, 5:

1. Stick to **1** sleep schedule.

2. Starting at **2**:00 p.m., eliminate all caffeine.

3. Stop alcohol **3** hours before bedtime.

4. Stop exercising **4** hours before bed.

5. Give the sun a high **5** every morning for 15 minutes.

1. Stick to 1 sleep schedule. When your sleep has a regular rhythm, your biological clock will be in sync and all your other bodily functions will go smoother, including sleep!

2. Starting at 2:00 p.m., eliminate all caffeine. Many of my patients admit that they can drink a cup of coffee and go straight to bed. In truth, however, even though your eyes are closed, the caffeine is stimulating your brain out of deep and REM sleep.

3. No alcohol within 3 hours of bedtime. While alcohol initially makes you sleepy, it also interferes with the deep stages of sleep. This recommendation is based on alcohol metabolism. Alcohol is metabolized at a rate of 0.015 of the blood alcohol level (BAL) per hour. Based on the height and weight of the average woman, when she has a BAL of 0.05, it will take about 3.3 hours for her to metabolize about three drinks.

Alcohol leads to fragmented sleep. It causes you to awaken more often in the second half of the night and makes it difficult to get back to sleep. And the closer to your bedtime that you drink, the more disturbed your sleep will be.

Alcohol's depressant effect on the central nervous system can also worsen preexisting sleep apnea by increasing muscular relaxation. Even in people who typically don't have sleep apnea, narrowing of the airway passages has been shown to occur when they've consumed moderate levels of alcohol before bedtime.[1] And even if apnea doesn't occur, there is a higher risk of snoring in those who drink alcohol before bedtime.

4. Stop exercising 4 hours before bed. Exercising during the day promotes better sleep. But exercising too close to bedtime makes many women feel wide awake and keyed up. Thirty minutes of vigorous aerobic exercise can also keep your body temperature elevated for about 4 hours, which can inhibit sleep (though the temperature drop after 4 hours can be helpful!).

5. Give the sun a high 5 every morning. Getting outside in the sun for 15 minutes each and every morning helps to regulate your production of melatonin, the sleep hormone, and reset your biological clock. This lets your body know it is time to wake up (and maybe even to smell the coffee!).

These rules are so central to the success of *The Sleep Doctor's Diet Plan* that they deserve to be examined in closer detail. They are very specific and work to virtually guarantee you a better night's sleep and subsequent weight loss. It's important to use the five rules together; adopting only one or two rules will not give you the benefit of better sleep and weight loss. However, after following the five rules daily, you will see a noticeable difference in your sleep quality, energy level, and weight.

Rule #1: Stick to 1 Sleep Schedule

Of all the sleep tips you could ever read or hear about, the most important one is to *stick to one sleep schedule—every day.* This means going to bed and waking up at the same time each day. When sleep has a regular rhythm, your biological clock will be in sync and all your other bodily functions will go more smoothly, including your sleep.

You are probably squirming as you read this, thinking about your own sleep issues and how you have anything *but* a regular sleep routine. To establish a sleep routine, there are some facts you need to know about yourself. For example, do you know how long you should sleep? *There is no one answer to this question that applies to everyone.* The National Sleep Foundation suggests that women aim for *between 7 and 8 hours* of sleep, and that is a good starting place. But some women are still sleepy even after 7 to 8 hours of sleep a night, while others thrive on 6.5 hours. How do you know how much sleep is right for you? Here's an exercise that can help you determine your optimal sleep number.

Figure Out *Your* Bedtime

When was the last time someone told you when to go to bed? Age 8 or 10, maybe? It turns out that going to bed at the right time is one of the most important factors in getting good sleep. Pick the right bedtime for you and stick to it. How do you know what this is? I have a formula that I give to my patients.

Sleep cycles are 90 minutes long, and the most satisfying sleep includes a set number of full cycles—ideally, five. If you multiply 5 and 90, it equals 450 minutes, or 7.5 hours. Since most of us have a wake-up time that's determined by kids or work, count backward *7.5 hours* from that wake-up time to find your real bedtime, the time when you should be turning off the lights. (For example, if you wake up at 7:30 a.m., it's lights out at midnight.) If you wake up a few minutes before your alarm, you have found your bedtime. If not, then try going to bed 20 minutes earlier each night until you find the right bedtime for you.

How Much Sleep Do You Really Need?

Let's assume that you have determined that you need 8 hours of sleep every night to feel rested. Throughout the course of the day you withdraw about 8 hours from your sleep bank account, generating a sleep debt (similar to an overdraft on your checking account). At night, as you snooze, you replenish your account by making regular deposits of z's. If your deposits keep pace with your withdrawals, all is well.

If, however, you sleep only 6.5 hours on a given night, you will still owe 1.5 hours to your sleep bank account. If you do this for 5 nights in a row, you will have lost almost an entire night's sleep! You will then need extra sleep over the next few days to replenish your sleep debt. But be warned: *Sometimes sleep debts get so large that you can't repay them entirely.* Note also that sleep is not something you can bank in advance; if you know you are going to be out late, you cannot get extra sleep for a few evenings prior to save up for a big night on the town. You can replenish some or most of your prior sleep debt, but you can't stockpile extra sleep for the future.

Now Calculate Your Sleep Debt

To see if you have a sleep debt, you need to check how long it takes you to fall asleep. *If you fall asleep in less than 5 minutes, you are probably sleep deprived!* This can indicate that your sleep debt is quite large. But this is not the only test, since some of my sleep-deprived patients have trouble falling asleep even though they are exhausted.

To figure out your sleep debt, start on a Friday evening. Now go to sleep at the same time for the next 6 nights. During this week, give yourself the opportunity to get 7 to 8 hours of uninterrupted sleep each night.

Then, on the next Saturday morning 1 week later, I want you to sleep in. See how long your body will let you sleep. If you sleep longer than you did during the week, then you can still have a sleep debt. That's a sign that you should get more sleep each night during the week.

If you cannot do this sleep debt exercise, try another simple task: See what time you awaken *without an alarm.* If you need an alarm to wake up, there is a good chance that you are sleep deprived and have a sleep debt.

Don't Miss Your Sleep Window

Have you ever been really hungry, only to have the hunger pangs disappear after an hour or so even though you haven't eaten anything? The same thing happens with sleep. You can be so tired at night that you can barely keep your eyes open, and then all of a sudden you get a second wind. What really happens is that you miss your window of opportunity for sleep, or your *sleep window.* Since you're not in bed or already asleep, your nervous system kicks in and gets you going again. Trying to sleep once you get that second wind is often a lesson in frustration. If you stick to your ideal bedtime, you will find that your sleep window will move to your bedtime!

This may take a while to happen. But I promise that finding your proper sleep window does work!

Stress-Tackling Tools for Maximum Weight Loss

When Jessica came to my clinic for help managing stress, she said that along with worries about income, job, and parenting, she also worried about her father, who was in his eighties and lived alone. This 43-year-old single mom lay awake each night wondering how she could possibly manage caregiving on top of her other job and home

HOW THE RELAXATION RESPONSE CAN HELP YOU SLEEP

The relaxation response helps decrease your levels of the stress hormones cortisol and adrenaline and boosts restful sleep.[2, 3] Relaxation techniques can trigger the relaxation response—a physiological state characterized by a feeling of warmth and quiet mental alertness. This is the opposite of the **fight-or-flight** response produced by stress. Once you learn how to use the relaxation response each night, bloodflow to your brain will increase, and your brain waves will shift from the alert beta rhythm to the relaxed alpha rhythm. Practiced regularly, the relaxation techniques in this chapter can counteract the debilitating effects of stress.

responsibilities. To cope, she would snack at night when her young daughter was asleep. Then she'd feel so guilty about eating too many chips and crackers that she would lie awake with one more big fat worry added to her long list.

I explained to Jessica that stress is the number one trigger of sleeplessness and sleeplessness was partially to blame for her weight gain. When you add up the stress Jessica had as a working single mom who was also caring for an aging parent, it was no wonder that she was overweight and in overload.

Jessica's sleeplessness resulting from her job-related worries is not an uncommon problem. In fact, after the US economic collapse began in 2008, studies showed that more than half of people polled reported physical and emotional symptoms as a result of stress, including feelings of fatigue and lying awake at night. Some studies showed that stress levels measured among working mothers often approached the stress levels of those involved in combat![4]

Single working women, including women who are single parents, like Jessica, and juggle kids and careers, are often greatly stressed by overwork, lack of time, and no energy. As anxieties and fears increase, symptoms such as more belly fat, elevated blood pressure, and faster heart rate can also worsen. With high anxiety, you have even more sleep issues and related weight issues. Plus, being tired after a poor night's sleep can make it hard to be effective at work or patient with family and friends.[5]

Caroline, 39, came to see me with the most common complaint I hear: "Dr. Breus, I don't sleep at all. When I get in the bed, I cannot turn my mind off, and I just lie there all night long, thinking of everything I need to do tomorrow and over the next few weeks. Before I know it, it is morning, and I dread the day."

I told her about an old trick I use that often helps people who repeatedly go over worries in their minds just before sleep. I asked Caroline to *count backward from 300 by 3s* while she was lying in bed. I have found that counting backward from 300 by 3s is so mathematically complicated that I cannot think of anything else and so boring that I fall right to sleep. Turns out that many of my patients do, too! It takes quite a bit of thinking to accomplish this, and you can't ruminate about anything else that's troubling you at the same time.

When Caroline returned 2 weeks later, she said that counting backward was difficult and had been more effective than she had expected. She felt in control of both her stress and her sleep. She was modifying her sleep schedule and had even lowered her caffeine intake. Caroline was also less frustrated and distressed about her sleep and starting to take things in stride instead of micromanaging her sleep style.

Women and Stress

Almost all the patients I see at my sleep clinic are like Jessica in that they have some type of emotional distress. In fact, most women end up crying during the session—not necessarily because they are sad, but because they are frustrated and exhausted from feeling too tired and too fat. These patients often think that they are sleep and diet failures. They tell themselves:

- Sleep is just so basic for most people that it must be my fault that I can't sleep.
- Diets are easy to follow, so it must be my fault that my weight won't budge.

Well, *they are wrong*; they did not *fail* at sleeping or dieting. They just need to make some changes to their lifestyles and sleep hygiene habits in order to clear their minds so they can relax and feel sleepy at bedtime. Then, by getting better and longer sleep, they can resolve their weight problems. I'd like to reiterate that all the sleep advice in the world won't help you if you have poor sleep hygiene habits, so you have to act with common sense about sleep, including:

- Going to bed at the same time every night
- Getting up at the same time every day (even on the weekends)
- Keeping your bedroom cool and comfortable
- Eating right and avoiding caffeinated drinks before bedtime
- Limiting alcohol, nicotine, and heavy meals before bedtime
- Exercising regularly
- Clearing your mind of stressful clutter

Keeping a **Worry Journal** can help ease your mind about stressful topics. Here's a sample entry.

- I have a million things to do tomorrow, and I am sure I will forget one!
  - **The Solution:** I am going to give myself 10 minutes now and 10 minutes in the morning to compile a list of what I can accomplish in the day. I'll write up a tentative schedule so I can get through my day efficiently.

DO YOU HAVE A FAMILY HISTORY OF SHORT SLEEPERS?

If you're a short sleeper, which is technically defined as someone who regularly gets fewer than 6 hours a night, are you living well off that brief sleep? Interestingly, recent research shows that some people are genetically predisposed to be short sleepers and function perfectly well on less than 6 hours a night.[6]

In one study, a researcher followed a woman and her mother—both of whom need only 5.5 hours of sleep each night—and, surprisingly, the women awoke feeling vibrant and refreshed in the morning. Genetic tests showed that the mother and daughter had a particular gene called **DEC2** that predisposed them to need less sleep.[7] Such people are probably genetic anomalies, somehow differently programmed to evade all the risks related to insufficient sleep. For them, 4 to 6 hours is sufficient. But before you assign yourself to this group and dismiss any thoughts of having a sleep deficit, know that these people are thought to number less than 0.1 percent of the population.

There are plenty of stories to go around about famous short sleepers. Those who have claimed to get by on only 4 hours of sleep include Jay Leno, Madonna, Martha Stewart, Margaret Thatcher, Michelangelo, Napoléon Bonaparte, Florence Nightingale, and Thomas Edison (whose invention of the lightbulb forever changed our sleep habits). Winston Churchill got by on 6 hours, and Leonardo da Vinci kept one of the most outrageously crazy sleep schedules ever, sleeping for 15 minutes every 4 hours, day and night.

The reality is that the vast majority of us need *plenty of sleep*. Just as you only occasionally hear about people who drank, smoked, and ate poorly living to the ripe old age of 100, neither do you hear about too many people who skimp on sleep and escape the associated physical and mental health problems. Those who claim they can get by on little sleep are likely fooling themselves. And ultimately, their bodies won't be fooled.

- I am concerned about Johnny's academic performance at school.

  - ○ **The Solution:** In the morning, I will make a list of my concerns about Johnny's school performance. Then, I will call the school and schedule a parent-teacher conference to see if he needs further help or if I'm just exaggerating the problem.

- My supervisor at work might think I forgot to attend to a task she assigned me.

  - ○ **The Solution:** Tomorrow I will write my supervisor an e-mail to let her know I completed the task. I will attach a copy of my work to the e-mail in case she hasn't had time to read it. Also, I will put a copy of it on her desk for future reference.

- I really want to lose weight, but I can't stop eating. Every time I think about dieting, it makes me want to eat more!

  - ○ **The Solution:** When I wake up, I'm going to clean out my kitchen and toss any food that's not in my diet plan. I'll write down the foods I can eat and tape the list to my kitchen cabinet. I'll schedule 15 minutes of exercise into my activities twice a day and try to go to bed an hour earlier to get more sleep.

Use the Sleep Doctor's Power-Down Hour™

The *Power-Down Hour* is a period of time that should immediately precede your bedtime. This time is important to allow your body and mind to get ready for sleep. It's important to understand that sleep does not have an on/off switch. It's more like pulling your foot off the gas pedal and slowly applying it to the brake pedal. To get great sleep, you have to wind down, relax, and feel drowsy. The more time you allow yourself to prepare for restful sleep, the better sleep you will get. The Power-Down Hour works like this.

1. Set your alarm clock (or better still, a second alarm clock so you won't have to reset the first for the morning) for an hour earlier than your ideal bedtime. For women who sleep 7.5 hours a night, this would be 8.5 hours before you must wake up (e.g., if lights-out is at 10:30 p.m., set your alarm for 9:30 p.m.).

2. When your alarm clock rings, go to your room and turn the alarm off and then begin your Power-Down Hour. This is a reminder trick I teach my patients who say, "The night gets away from me, and I look up and it's midnight!"

3. Spend 20 minutes on things that must be done for tomorrow (packing lunches, setting out clothes, writing reminders—but no e-mail or computer work).

4. Spend 20 minutes on hygiene (washing face, brushing teeth, taking a hot shower or bath—*all done in dim lighting; remember, bright light reduces melatonin production*).

5. Spend 20 minutes relaxing or meditating in your bed in the dark. Don't forget to reset your alarm for morning, if necessary, as you prepare to crawl into bed.

Rule #2: Starting at 2:00 p.m., Eliminate All Caffeine

I know what you're thinking: Is he serious? How can stopping my caffeine intake at 2:00 p.m. help me lose weight? It's simple! Caffeine has what's called a half-life of about 8 hours, which means that its level is reduced but still somewhat effective in your system after this time. Caffeine is a stimulant, and it will prevent you from either falling asleep or having good sleep. *Remember, sleep helps you lose weight!*

"But I love my lattes and diet colas!" I hear you pleading.

Of course you do! But many insomniacs and disordered sleepers struggle with all-out addictions to caffeinated drinks. The need for caffeine creates a catch-22: If you don't sleep well at night, you're tired during the day and drink caffeinated drinks to stay awake and alert; this then impairs your ability to sleep at night. That is why this diet does not ask you to eliminate caffeine altogether, just to abstain from it in any form after 2:00 p.m.

My patient Lynn, 41, had an enormous sleep debt that made it hard for her to perform well at her job. Her weight was about 12 pounds higher than she preferred, and she felt nervous and on edge much of the time.

I asked Lynn to keep a Sleep Diary and to keep track of what she ate and drank and any medications she took.

When she showed me her Sleep Diary at the next visit, I was surprised to see that her caffeine intake was relatively normal (1 large cup of drip-brewed coffee in the morning). But in addition to her morning coffee, she was taking an OTC headache remedy that had a combination of acetaminophen and caffeine. While the amount of caffeine in each headache tablet (65 mg) was less than that in 1 cup of coffee, Lynn was taking the recommended two tablets (130 mg of caffeine) every 4 hours throughout the day, even right before bedtime at 11:00 p.m. This was like having a cup of strong brewed coffee every 4 hours! Caffeine can stay in your system for as long as 14 hours and, by increasing the number of times you awaken at night, decrease the total amount of sleep time.

Working together with her primary care doctor, Lynn got a full medical evaluation and a new headache treatment that was caffeine free. Within days, she began to see a dramatic improvement in her sleep quality, a greater ability to stay focused on her work, and even a reduction in her daily headaches. Perhaps the most impressive outcome was that she lost 6 pounds in 1 month without making any dietary changes.

It's true that caffeine boosts your energy for a little while as it blocks sleep-inducing chemicals in the brain and increases the production of adrenaline. Interestingly, caffeine also increases dopamine levels in the same way that amphetamines do. Dopamine is a neurotransmitter that activates the pleasure centers in certain parts of your brain. It is suspected that the dopamine connection is what's behind caffeine addiction. But when you depend on caffeine day after day for your "supercharge," your sleep (and your weight) will pay a steep price for this addiction. As anyone who's tried to cut out caffeine cold turkey knows, withdrawal symptoms can be difficult to unbearable, bringing headaches, fatigue, irritability, concentration problems, and sometimes even flulike symptoms such as nausea, muscle aches, and vomiting. I'll show you an easier way to withdraw from caffeine on page 110.

Warning: Energy Drinks Steal Your Sleep and Sanity

No longer targeted only at athletes, energy drinks became an enormous market as they found their way into the everyday lives of many Americans. Funny how energy drinks first emerged on the scene as dietary supplements; now we recognize that they are merely revved-up versions of soda.

There's a growing movement to require warning labels on energy drinks that contain large amounts of caffeine (yes, more than coffee in some cases) as a result of researchers' findings on these high-octane beverages.[8] The industry, of course, doesn't want to reveal much information about its products.

You may be surprised to learn that although the FDA limits the caffeine content of soft drinks to 71 mg per 12 fluid ounces, there's no limit on caffeine in energy drinks. And between the lack of information on most labels and the lack of regulation, it can be hard to know what's in an energy drink. That said, I believe the names of popular energy drinks give good hints about what their contents are. For best results for rest and weight loss, choose an energy drink that gets its energy boosting properties from vitamins and minerals, not sugar and caffeine. See my recommendations at www.theinsomniablog.com.

4 STEPS TO CUTTING BACK ON ENERGY DRINKS

Energy drinks can serve a constructive purpose in our lives when they're used appropriately. But the problem is that these drinks have become so mainstream that most people drink them indiscriminately. Along with their high caffeine content, energy drinks also contain a lot of sugar, which can add pounds to your frame and also disrupt a good night's sleep (which makes it harder to lose the weight).

Even people accustomed to limiting their coffee consumption in the latter parts of the day may inadvertently compromise their sleep with energy drinks. These energy bombs do more than work against sleep; they can cause you to feel anxious, jittery, wired, and tired all at the same time.

If you are hooked on energy drinks, you'll find that these four steps will help you eliminate them from your life—and in doing so, your sleep, weight loss, and natural energy will improve.

Step #1: Opt for a cup of plain black tea or coffee instead of waking up to a sugar-laden energy drink.

Step #2: Instead of having another energy drink at lunch, try a glass of unsweetened iced black or green tea. Again, drink water to replenish.

Step #3: Get over the late-afternoon hump with a protein-rich snack that has some carbohydrates. Try sliced turkey on whole wheat crackers or a scoop of nut butter and celery sticks. Also, get outside and get some sunlight, which will help regulate your production of melatonin. Spending some time outside in the sun will stop the pineal gland in your brain from producing melatonin, which is one reason you feel so sleepy.

Step #4: Avoid all sources of caffeine after *2:00 p.m.*

3 Easy Steps to Curtail Your Caffeine Addiction

Regular caffeine intake is linked to disturbed sleep and the daytime sleepiness that results from it.[9] If you need to cut back on caffeine, here are three easy steps to help you.

Step #1: Consume caffeine as you normally do for a week while keeping a precise log of when you ingest anything that contains caffeine, as well as how much of it. Include items such as chocolate, tea, and caffeinated sodas and headache pills.

Step #2: At the end of the week, start reducing your caffeine intake little by little by eliminating the equivalent of ½ cup of coffee (40 mg of caffeine) a day. *Start with end-of-the-day caffeinated beverages.* Remember to have reduced- or zero-caffeine substitutes (such as decaf hot chocolate or herbal tea) on hand for those times of day when you're accustomed to drinking caffeinated beverages.

Step #3: When you can tolerate that lesser amount of caffeine, start replacing some of the other caffeinated drinks with lower-caffeine drinks such as tea.

Black tea has about 40 to 60 mg of caffeine per cup (about half the caffeine of 1 cup of coffee and carbonated caffeinated drinks like Coke and Pepsi). Black tea is also easier on the digestive system and rich in antioxidants, which can help prevent cancer and heart disease. Avoid adding sugar to teas and other caffeine substitutes. This only adds calories and causes upheavals in your blood glucose level, spiking it initially but then making it fall so low that you will be ravenous.

Other tips to help you cut back on caffeine:

- Watch out for hidden sources of caffeine, such as chocolate, medications, and frozen desserts.
- Cut off caffeine 8 hours before bedtime (e.g., at 2:00 p.m.).
- If you need caffeine late in the day, try to get it from a less potent source, like green tea, which has about 20 mg of caffeine.

- Try to regulate your caffeine intake by drinking the most highly caffeinated beverages in the early part of the day and then moving to less-caffeinated beverages.
  - Coffee in the morning
  - Tea or soda for lunch
  - Slightly caffeinated beverage before 2:00 p.m.
  - Water and other caffeine-free drinks such as herbal teas from 2:00 p.m. until bedtime
- Also remember that caffeine is a diuretic (it makes your body lose water), so when you indulge, you need to replenish fluid by drinking as much water as you can.
- If coffee is your beverage of choice, consider changing to a half-and-half blend of decaffeinated and caffeinated beans.
  - Drink your coffee *black*. Cream and sugar just add calories.

Rule #3: No Alcohol within 3 Hours of Bedtime

For years sleep researchers have known that *alcohol is the number one sleep aid in the world.* If you look back at the results of the 2005 *Sleep in America* poll, you will find that 11 percent of those polled used alcohol as a sleep aid at least a few nights a week.[10] Another study conducted in the Detroit area showed that 13 percent of those polled had used alcohol as a sleep aid in the past year.[11]

And alcohol is *not* the answer to getting better sleep. While alcohol can make you sleepy, it also does the following to detract from sound sleep.

- Keeps you from reaching the deep stages of sleep
- Dehydrates you
- Awakens you in the middle of the night (usually to go to the bathroom)

Having a few drinks before bedtime will increase your NREM sleep (Stages 1 and 2) and reduce your REM sleep. You'll remember that REM sleep helps you organize and store memories. Too little REM sleep can be devastating for the brain and body. In addition, REM sleep is the sleep stage during which the most calories are burned. And alcohol is filled with empty calories, so drinking is never a good idea when you're trying to lose weight.

Don't get me wrong. Having a glass of red wine with dinner is fine and may be healthful. Some studies indicate that the antioxidants in red wine may have some health benefits. Why have I chosen to prohibit alcohol intake 3 hours before bed? Simple. To account for the rate of metabolism. Alcohol is metabolized at a rate of 0.015 of your blood alcohol level per hour. So if you have a blood alcohol level of 0.05, it will take you 3.3 hours to metabolize it all and then eliminate it through urination. Your height and weight determine how many drinks this is for you.

Many people who rely on alcohol for sleep report multiple awakenings and shallow sleep. Some also experience vivid nightmares, night sweats, and inability to relax. So it is simply a bad idea to have alcohol in your system while you're sleeping.

Rule #4: Stop Exercising 4 Hours before Bed

No one would argue that exercise isn't good for you. It keeps muscles and bones strong and maintains good cardiovascular health. You know that exercise boosts your metabolism, which is important for weight loss. But do you understand the immense benefits exercise provides in enhancing your sleep quality? Many of my sleep patients who lead sedentary lives and don't exercise regularly are missing out on an excellent sleep remedy. Data suggest not only that exercising during the day will help you fall asleep more quickly and plunge you into deeper sleep for a longer period of time, but also that exercising causes your body to produce growth hormones, which help it to repair and revitalize itself. Many of my patients report that they sleep better with regular exercise and that they feel more alert and rejuvenated the following day.

Studies show that exercise and physical activity (especially when done outside in the early morning light) help to regulate the circadian rhythm, which is vital to making you feel sleepy at bedtime. But it's best to avoid exercise right before bedtime, especially if physical activity keys and warms you up. After 30 minutes of cardiovascular exercise, your core body temperature will have risen based on how vigorously you worked out. It generally takes about 4 hours for your temperature to fall, which signals to the brain to get ready for sleep. Core body temperature has a 24-hour rhythm that supplies the internal timing for sleep and wakefulness. Sleep typically occurs when your temperature is declining, whereas wakefulness occurs when your temperature is rising.

So, as in most things in life . . . *timing is everything!*

Can Late-Day Exercise Boost Sleep?

If you are ultrasensitive to stress, moderate exercise performed several hours before bedtime can help you to sleep better. Exercising—especially outdoors in the natural light—is a healthy way to boost sleep as opposed to resorting to sleep aids, alcohol, or other possibly harmful substances.

Another benefit of exercising in the late afternoon or early evening is linked to the reduced secretion of stress hormones after exercise. It's been found that women with insomnia tend to stay hyperaroused by the increased levels of stress hormones in their blood. These women are abnormally sensitive to stress, which then wreaks havoc with their thoughts, causing them to ruminate and be on high alert at night instead of sleeping.

While exercise will increase production of stress hormones for a short time after a workout, several hours later these hormones drop to low levels—lower than they were before exercising. The timing of this drop again demonstrates the benefits of late afternoon/early evening exercise, particularly for women who are sensitive to stress.

The Science behind Exercise and Sleep

Scientists theorize in what they call the thermogenic hypothesis that exercise promotes sleep by slightly elevating the body's temperature. Because the core temperature drops in the afternoon, exercising during that time will raise it and increase alertness. This helps to explain why late afternoon is the ideal time to exercise for some women *(just don't exercise 4 hours or less before bed!)*.

Say you exercise for at least 20 to 30 minutes. This physical activity increases your body temperature, which stays elevated for about 4 hours (depending upon the type and duration of exercise). Once your body cools down, your temperature actually drops to about 1°F lower than your normal resting temperature! This small drop in body temperature may be exactly what helps you get a good night's sleep by signaling your brain to release melatonin.

I read a revealing report from researchers at the Federal University of São Paulo in Brazil who investigated this relationship between exercise and sleep. In the study, 60 patients (including 28 women) with chronic primary insomnia were divided into four different groups. Three of the groups were told to exercise and then had their sleep analyzed in a sleep lab. One group, the moderate exercisers, ran on a treadmill at an easy pace for 50 minutes. Another group, the heavy exercisers, ran in three intense 10-minute bursts, with 10-minute breaks in between. The third group focused on strength training for 50 minutes, using both upper- and lower-body muscles. The final group was a control group that did not exercise.

Upon analyzing everyone's sleep quality, researchers found no significant changes in that of the nonexercisers, the heavy exercisers, or the strength trainers. But get this! *The participants who exercised at a moderate pace were able to get to sleep faster, sleep longer, and stay asleep most of the night.*[12]

The applications of this particular study are limited because it looked at only 1 night of sleep after exercise. Still, I think it is extremely promising that sleep doctors are discovering more natural solutions to help people sleep better.

Be Your Own Sleep Lab

The secret to getting the best sleep benefits from exercise is to know when the best time to exercise is and what the right type of exercise is. *Experiment with exercise and sleep to see what works best for you.* Does late-afternoon or early evening exercise give you the restful sleep that you are seeking? If not, try exercising in the morning, especially outdoors, so your circadian rhythms can benefit from the early morning light.

Finding the perfect time to exercise and the perfect kind and amount of exercise can seem overwhelming. However, to discover the best time for and duration of exercise, try these very simple steps.

1. **First, see your doctor.** Visit your health care provider to make sure you are healthy and can begin an exercise program.
2. **Keep an exercise journal.** A spiral notebook will work well, or you can track your workouts on your mobile device. Use your journal to record your daily exercise regimen along with any noticeable changes in your sleep patterns that accompany this new routine.
3. **Start exercising!** Try morning exercise if that feels right for you— or try late-afternoon/early evening exercise. Attempt to exercise at the same time of day for at least 5 days a week for 2 weeks and then rate your sleep. Then, switch it up. If you were exercising in the afternoon, move your workouts to the morning or vice versa. See if you notice any sleep-quality changes. Which exercise time works best to help you get great sleep?
4. **Aim for endurance.** Get at least 30 minutes of moderate cardio exercise on most days of the week. Afterward, stretch. Take a yoga class or perform some of your favorite feel-good stretches. Looser muscles allow for a better night's rest.

FIND YOUR FAVORITE ACTIVITIES TO BOOST GOOD SLEEP

Choose the activities you enjoy from the following list and work out more to improve your sleep quality.

Low Intensity (Good for those who have a sedentary lifestyle)

Ballroom dancing (slow)

Bowling

Golf (using a cart)

Tai chi

Water aerobics (slow)

Yoga

Moderate Intensity (Good for those who are moderately fit)

Aerobics (low impact)

Badminton

Ballroom dancing (fast)

Biking (moderate)

Elliptical trainer

Gardening

Golf (walking)

Mall walking (moderate pace)

Stair climbing

Stationary biking

Swimming (moderate)

Tennis (doubles)

Walking (brisk)

Water aerobics

High Intensity (Good for those who are aerobically fit)

Aerobics (high impact)

Basketball

Biking (hills)

Dancing (fast)

Hiking

Jogging

Jumping rope

Karate

Kickboxing

Rollerblading

Running

Soccer

Spinning (ultra-intensity indoor cycling)

Swimming (fast)

Tennis (singles)

Rule #5: Give the Sun a High 5 Every Morning

Getting outside in the sun for 15 minutes each morning helps to regulate the production of melatonin, the sleep hormone. Your internal body clock (the circadian rhythm) runs on a 24-hour schedule and functions best when you are exposed to a regular pattern of light and dark. Malfunctions in your circadian rhythms because of changes in light and dark exposure can negatively impact your ability to get a good night's sleep.

Unfortunately, unlike our cave-dwelling ancestors who rose with the sun and retired with the moon, most of us let the demands of everyday life dictate the times for sleeping and rising. Millions of women today force their bodies to adjust to artificial sleep schedules, negatively affecting both their sleep and their health.

For instance, shift workers who sleep when their natural biological clocks tell them to be awake are at an increased risk for illness, including stress disorders. Sleeping in opposition to your body clock affects the production of melatonin, which is essential for starting and maintaining sleep. In addition, other body cycles, such as the rise and fall of body temperature and the ebb and flow of certain hormones, are affected by changes in light and dark.

If you're a sound sleeper and these systems are all working in sync, sleep is easy! Chances are you feel rested and don't even need an alarm clock to wake up each day. But if you're an ultrasensitive or anxious sleeper, your normal sleep-wake schedule and sleep quality can be greatly affected. Saluting the sun every morning can help you set your clock to the right time.

The Science behind Light and Sleep

Research has shown that exposure to morning light and evening light can have profound effects on circadian rhythms. For instance, in the shorter, darker days of winter, especially in the northernmost states, women often become depressed as a result of the decrease in sunlight. In the absence of daily bright light at the right time, hormones can be released at the wrong times of day. This causes the circadian rhythms to go awry, and negative mood symptoms can result.

Even a small amount of light exposure in the evening (like when you take off your makeup or turn on the light when using the bathroom at

2:00 a.m.) can cause your brain to think that morning has come. Once the light signals the brain to stop producing melatonin, you will have difficulty falling asleep again.

Light Therapy May Help Insomniacs

Insomnia (see page 33) is a sleep disorder characterized by having problems falling asleep, waking up frequently throughout the night, or awakening in the early morning and not being able to fall back to sleep. Many sleep experts believe that exposure to bright early morning or late-evening light can help insomniacs whose sleep problems might have a biological basis. It is important to know that night owls benefit from light therapy in the early morning hours and early birds in the evening. As with any alternative treatment, be sure to consult your physician or a sleep specialist before trying light therapy to help insomnia.

The Science behind Light, Sleep, and Weight Loss

While vitamin D is commonly known to build stronger bones, did you know that it might also help with weight loss? Findings show that most of us don't get enough vitamin D, and people who are overweight or obese may be at greater risk for low levels of this vitamin because body fat holds on to vitamin D, making it unavailable for use by the rest of the body. Furthermore, a low serum level of vitamin D inhibits production of leptin (the "stop eating" hormone). And since it's thought that overweight people are less active, which means they *spend less time* in the sun (which makes your body produce vitamin D), they both make less vitamin D and have less of what they do produce available to their bodies. The result is that they don't have enough vitamin D to produce enough leptin to tell them to stop eating.[13]

Some new studies[14] also link a low level of vitamin D to *mood disorders such as mild depression and to weight gain.* In fact, some psychiatrists treat seasonal affective disorder (SAD) with vitamin D. SAD causes low mood and feelings of depression, hypersomnolence, carbohydrate craving, weight gain, and loss of libido during the fall and winter. Usually starting at about age 23, SAD is more common in women than in men and affects about 6 percent of Americans. Because the lack of sufficient daylight during winter months partially causes SAD, we seldom find it in countries within 30 degrees of the equator, where the days and nights are of nearly equal length all year round. Many findings have been published about the biochemical mechanisms behind this disorder, including circadian phase conditions, abnormal melatonin secretion, and problems with serotonin synthesis.[15]

Researchers have known for many years that when light strikes the human retina, the pineal gland is stimulated via nerve pathways. This stimulation decreases its secretion of melatonin. This suggests that melatonin is related to depression in people with SAD and that light therapy has an antidepressant effect because it modifies the amount of melatonin in the nervous system. Other findings indicate that the neurotransmitter serotonin is involved in SAD and is affected by therapeutic light therapy.[16]

In one study, researchers gave vitamin D supplements to women who had low serum vitamin D levels and depressive symptoms. The supplementation was linked with an increase in serum vitamin D levels and a decline in low mood.[17]

Be Your Own Sleep Lab

Are you getting enough morning light? Follow these suggestions to up your light quotient.

- Have your window shades open at night so you can get some morning sun (assuming that there is not enough light at night to keep you awake).
- Consider getting a dawn-simulating device or clock.
- Walk your pet right when you wake up. That way you get your exercise and sunlight.

- Make sure you shower in a well-lit bathroom or, better yet, one with natural sunlight.
- Have your bed face a window that faces east so you can catch the sunrise.
- Have your breakfast outside, weather permitting.
- Avoid wearing sunglasses for your first 15 minutes outside (only with your doctor's permission).

If your schedule or other circumstances make getting true morning sun difficult for you, you can try working with a simulated source of daylight. Historically, researchers have used light therapy with patients who have sleep issues and/or SAD.[18] With light therapy, the person sits about 2 feet away from a very bright light, usually a 10,000-lux light box (about 20 times brighter than normal room lighting), for a 45- to 60-minute session per day. If the symptoms do not resolve, twice-daily sessions are tried. Individuals who respond to light therapy are encouraged to continue with it until they can be out in the springtime sun again.

Recently there has been an important discovery regarding light therapy. Since scientists identified a particular receptor in the eye, they have found that when light at a certain frequency is used in therapy, the light's intensity can be lessened to about 3,000 lux and sessions shortened to only 20 minutes. The frequency is that of a *blue light*.[19] There are commercially available light-therapy boxes that provide this particular light intensity, and this is the type of light therapy I use in my practice.

Light-therapy boxes are available on the Internet. If you want to purchase one, select one that provides a blue light with a frequency of between 460 and 480 nanometers. Make sure the light-therapy box has been approved by a doctor and has specific guidelines for helping with your particular sleep problem. Generally, I ask my patients to use a light-therapy schedule that I provide based on their particular problems.

Try this bright, early morning light therapy for several weeks. If you notice no improvement in your sleep-wake schedule in that time, then consult a sleep specialist.

THE STORY ABOUT INSOMNIA AND ACUPUNCTURE

In a recent review of the literature (2009), researchers looked at 46 randomized trials with 3,811 patients and determined that acupuncture is an effective treatment for insomnia. More specifically, the meta-analysis showed that acupuncture was more effective than nothing, and more effective than a sham acupressure. Acupuncture and medication appear to be more effective than just medication alone, and acupuncture with herbs was more effective than herbs alone. While an interesting review, unfortunately the findings did not give an indication as to which specific acupuncture points were effective for sleep.[20]

Ancient Therapies to New Age Trends

Along with the *Sleep Doctor's 5 Simple Rules,* there are some ancient therapies and New Age trends that I also recommend to my patients to increase their relaxation at bedtime. Over the past several decades, certain ancient practices of peoples of Eastern countries such as China and India have been adopted in the American culture. This is especially true for relaxation techniques.

The regular practice of yoga can help you relax your body and mind, as can listening to some types of slow, rhythmic music. Also, deep abdominal breathing and progressive muscle relaxation are excellent mind–body exercises to help you focus on the moment and remove the effects of daily stressors that keep you wound up at night.

Ease Tension with Yoga

Yoga is a fundamental part of ayurvedic medicine, India's traditional system of medicine. Yoga not only reduces anxiety, but also promotes overall well-being and helps achieve mind–body balance.

Yoga originated as an Eastern practice, but Westerners have flocked to it in droves, particularly *hatha yoga,* which focuses on poses called postures. Practitioners of yoga find that this ancient discipline helps to relieve stress, promote deep relaxation, connect the mind and body, and aid with sleep problems.[21]

Because yoga is a type of mind–body therapy, the postures are designed to stretch the mind and body beyond their normal limits and then bring them together to act in unison again. Yoga postures can relieve mild aches and pains, menstrual cramps, and lower-back pain. By using deep breathing and concentration techniques in conjunction with poses, you learn to calm your mind and increase your flexibility, coordination, and strength.

Pranayama, the conscious focus on and control of breath to heal disease, is an important part of yoga. Breath exercises performed along with different yoga postures can increase blood circulation.

You do not have to study for years to enjoy some of yoga's healing benefits. Find a local yoga studio and take a class or two. In addition, try this 15-minute routine with a few simple poses before bedtime.

- **Bedtime Cat Stretch with Child's Pose (5 minutes)**
    1. Get on your hands and knees with your spine straight, your palms under your shoulders, and your knees under your hips. Let the tops of your feet rest on the floor.
    2. As you inhale, relax your abs. Lengthen through your spine as you lift your head toward the ceiling and let your belly drop toward the floor. Return to the original position.
    3. Exhale as you drop your head toward the floor, round your back toward the ceiling, and pull your belly toward your spine.
    4. Extend your arms out in front of you on the floor and settle your hips on your heels. Let your forehead drop to the floor to quiet your mind and relax your back even more. This is called child's pose.
    5. Return to the first position and slowly repeat both poses several times, until your back feels stretched out and your mind is relaxed.

- **Rock-a-Bye Roll (3 minutes)**
  1. Lie on your back and hug your knees to your chest.
  2. Cross your ankles and if you can, wrap both arms around your shins.
  3. Inhale as you take 3 seconds to slowly rock yourself forward and then exhale as you take 3 seconds to rock back. Do this 10 times.

- **Nighttime Goddess Stretch (2 minutes)**
  1. Lie on your back with your knees bent.
  2. Put the soles of your feet together and let your knees fall open to form a diamond shape with your legs.
  3. Rest your arms by your sides in the most comfortable position you can find.
  4. If you feel any strain, put small pillows under your knees to elevate them.

- **Corpse Pose (5 minutes)**
  1. Lie on your back on a comfortable surface. Keep your arms on the floor by your sides and your legs extended naturally from your hips. (Your feet will be about 12 inches apart and your toes turned outward slightly, because your feet, ankles, and legs will be relaxed.)
  2. With your palms facing up, move your hands and arms outward, to about 8 to 10 inches from your body. Lengthen your back on the floor and feel all of your muscles stretching and releasing.
  3. Notice your shoulder blades and hips and distribute your weight evenly on both sides of your body. Adjust the position until you feel balanced on both sides.
  4. Scan your muscles for any tension and consciously relax every muscle group, including your throat, face, and eye muscles. Continue this conscious scanning as you continue to relax.
  5. As you lie there, feel your breathing take you into a deeper, more relaxed state.

Deep Abdominal Breathing

Deep abdominal breathing oxygenates the brain, helps to end the stress cycle, and enables the heart rate and blood pressure to return to normal levels. Breathing deeply in this way also releases morphinelike pain relievers called *endorphins* and *enkephalins* that are associated with happy, positive feelings. During deep abdominal breathing, you add extra oxygen to the blood and decrease the release of stress hormones.

Here's how to practice deep abdominal breathing before bedtime.

1. While lying in bed, place your hands on your abdomen and take in a slow, deliberate, deep breath through your nostrils. If your hands are rising and your abdomen is expanding, then you are breathing correctly. If your hands do not rise but you see your chest rising, you are breathing incorrectly. Focus on your belly, and even slowly push your belly out until you get used to doing this breathing exercise.

2. Inhale to a count of 5, pause for 3 seconds, and then exhale to a count of 5. Start with 8 repetitions of this exercise and then gradually add more until you are doing 15.

Progressive Muscle Relaxation

Progressive muscle relaxation (PMR) is a technique that changes your physical and emotional responses to stress. PMR involves contracting and then relaxing all the major muscle groups in the body, beginning with the head and then proceeding to the neck, arms, chest, back, belly, pelvis, legs, and feet. One way to use this for stress reduction is to do it before you get out of bed in the morning and again before you close your eyes to sleep at night. Studies show that volunteers who practice PMR experience significant dips in heart rate and levels of perceived stress and of cortisol, the stress hormone that increases in response to sleep deprivation. It's harder to sleep when your cortisol level is high, plus a high level can increase your appetite and result in weight gain.

To do PMR:

1. Find a comfortable, quiet place where you will not be disturbed. I ask my patients to try this exercise while lying in bed and to allow about 15 minutes for it.

2. Start by tensing the muscles of the head to the count of 7 and then releasing them to the count of 7.

3. Perform deep abdominal breathing (see the opposite page) as you do PMR, breathing in while you tense the muscles and breathing out while you relax them.

For some patients, I recommend doing the deep breathing exercise prior to PMR, just to get their bodies ready for true relaxation.

Imagine Yourself Sleeping Peacefully

Visualization (or guided imagery) is a natural stress-release activity that you can do wherever you are, at any time of the day or night. I have found this relaxation exercise to be particularly helpful for people when they wake up in the middle of the night. By using visualization, you can allow your imagination to take over as you focus on your senses to create the desired state of relaxation in your mind.

1. **Lie on your back in a comfortable position.** Prop pillows under your knees to take pressure off your back. If this is still uncomfortable, sit in a chair with good back support. Close your eyes and take several deep breaths.

2. **Imagine a peaceful place.** This might be somewhere you've visited, giving you a mental picture of it. Perhaps this is the seashore at sunset or sunrise, a mountain cabin next to a babbling brook,

or you floating on a raft on a lake on a sunny day. Make sure your "peaceful place" is serene and relaxing; try to recall all the details of this place.

3. **Continue to breathe deeply and slowly as you keep this image in your mind.** Imagine all the stress, worries, and tension leaving your body. Feel the air temperature at your special place. See the colors surrounding you. What sounds do you hear? Smell the freshness of the air. Touch the gentleness of the moment. Take in all the sensory details of your relaxing place and continue to de-stress.

4. **After about 15 minutes, slowly open your eyes and reacclimatize yourself to the room.** Stretch your arms and legs; gently turn your head from side to side and feel the tension release. Carry the calm feeling you now have with you through the day.

Once you have tried visualization a few times and gotten the hang of it, it is a tool you can use upon awakening during the night. Some of my patients are able to imagine their peaceful place and within minutes, they gently drift back to sleep.

Calm Anxiety with Meditation

Meditation is a commonly used ayurvedic therapy that helps put the mind and body into a state of relaxation. Meditating quietly each day can ease anxiety for some people.

With meditation, you focus your mind on one thought, phrase, or prayer for a certain period of time. Meditation allows you to purposefully pay attention to what is happening in the present moment without being distracted by what has already happened or what might happen. This leads to the relaxation response, which decreases your heart rate, blood pressure, respiratory rate, and muscle tension, all of which aid in the process of sleep. Meditation also decreases secretion of stress hormones such as cortisol and adrenaline.

Meditation can guide you beyond the negative thoughts and agitations of the busy mind and allow you to become "unstuck" from fear and other disturbing emotions. When you learn how to meditate

COPING WITH TRAVEL AND SLEEP

When you will be traveling, it's important to plan ahead in order to cope with sleep disruptions such as too much light in the hotel room and time changes. Here are some tips.

1. **Ask for a hotel room that faces west,** since the sun rises in the east and is likely to awaken you earlier than necessary. Also request that it be a corner room away from elevators and vending machines.

2. **Exercise while you're on the road.** Studies show that exercise and physical activity (especially that done outside in the early morning light) help regulate the circadian rhythm, which is vital to feeling sleepy at bedtime. But avoid exercise right before bedtime if physical activity keys you up. Sometimes exercise can be stimulating and keep you from falling asleep.

3. **Get solid sleep the night before the trip.** Showing up at important business meetings sleep deprived is not a good way to start your trip. A study showed that sleep deprivation the night before travel had the biggest effect on performance. And if you have poor job performance, you can count on poor sleep to follow.

4. **Pack** your favorite pillow, earplugs, a sleep mask, and a clip for the drapes. These devices are particularly helpful for women who have difficulty sleeping in new environments.

5. **Avoid alcohol.** While drinking a cocktail or a glass of wine before bedtime may help you relax and fall asleep, alcohol can also create sleep disturbances.

6. **Bring along a meditation or relaxation CD to help you unwind before bed.** Or, if possible, get a room with a tub and take a hot bath or shower before bed.

effectively, you will be able to switch into this relaxation state at will. To learn to meditate, try the following:

1. Sit in a comfortable chair in a quiet room. Make sure there are no distractions. Close your eyes as you begin to meditate.
2. Focus your attention on the silent or whispered repetition of a word, sound, phrase, or prayer. Other alternatives are to focus on the sensation of each breath or to imagine a space that is white and empty.
3. Every time you notice that your attention has wandered (which will occur naturally), gently redirect your thoughts back without judging yourself. If you continue to practice this, you will learn how to do meditation correctly.

Meditation can take years to master, but the good news is that you don't have to be a master. With practice, this natural therapy can help you relax and fall asleep quickly. You might combine meditation with deep abdominal breathing and progressive muscle relaxation to help you "unplug" before bedtime.

Try a Self-Massage to Boost Sleepiness

Some women who find themselves too keyed up to fall asleep find that regular massages increase relaxation, which can help calm anxiety and improve sleep problems. Studies show that massage increases the production of endorphins.[22] These brain chemicals improve relaxation, relieve pain, and reduce panic and anxiety. Massage therapy also triggers the release of serotonin, the brain chemical that makes you feel calm and relaxed. When stress is alleviated, you can sleep peacefully.

You don't have to get a professional massage to benefit from touch therapy. If you have tension in your neck, shoulders, wrists, or other areas, you can massage the muscles gently with your fingers to loosen them, or you can ask your partner to do it. Here are more tips.

1. Gently rub a few drops of your favorite massage oil into the skin on the back of your neck. Use lavender massage oil to boost relaxation.
2. As you make contact with the skin, make a circular motion with your fingertips and move up and down your neck.
3. Work your way outward and down the sides of your neck to your shoulders, continuing the circular motion.
4. Squeeze each shoulder with the opposite hand one at a time. Then, using long strokes with your fingertips, gently sweep the skin from your neck to your shoulder and down to your elbow.
5. While self-massage is great, getting your spouse to give you a massage is even better. Do not be shy about asking for a massage, especially if it helps you sleep. But be warned, massage can be a form of foreplay, and when it leads to sex, it may energize rather than relax you.

Chill Out Naturally with Music

We know that music has a significant effect on respiration rate and anxiety level. In fact, at least one study has shown that certain musical forms can transport the listener's brain into an *alpha wave–generating* state of relaxation that is much like meditation.[23]

Music-assisted relaxation, in which music is combined with a relaxation technique, has been shown in clinical research to benefit sleep quality. In fact, a study at Case Western Reserve University showed that listening to music with 60 to 80 beats per minute for 45 minutes before bedtime improved perceived sleep quality, lengthened sleep duration, shortened the time it took to fall asleep, and resulted in more time asleep.[24] Another recent review paper concluded that music-assisted relaxation has a moderate positive effect on sleep quality and no side effects.[25] In still another pilot study, a "sleep system" of music improved perceived sleep quality, and, after being presented with the music twice during the same night, some participants had a slight increase in deep sleep.[26]

The current thoughts of sleep specialists about music therapy and sleep include:

1. Music before bed causes a relaxation response that makes falling asleep easier, and using a sound-masking machine at night might contribute to better sleep quality and fewer awakenings.

2. Music coupled with deep abdominal breathing (see page 124), a relaxation technique that many of us do without being aware of it, increases relaxation and decreases the time needed to fall asleep.

3. Music with a particular beat or sound wave forces the brain to "tune itself" (like a tuning fork) to the same wave.

SNOOZE YOU CAN USE: THE BEST MUSIC FOR SLEEP

- Consider purchasing music whose packaging says it has a particular number of beats (e.g., 60 to 80) per minute.
- Select music that is relaxing and make sure you enjoy the artist, or you may not listen to it. For instance, my patient Deb listens to Vivaldi's *The Four Seasons* before bedtime and visualizes scenes from the time she spent traveling throughout Italy. Another client, Karen, prefers Beethoven's *Moonlight Sonata*, while a third, Beth, finds that anything by Crosby, Stills and Nash helps to prepare her mind for sleep.

If you don't enjoy listening to music, try listening to sounds of the surf or thunderstorms to trigger thoughts of natural settings. Relaxation tapes and CDs with nature sounds can be purchased at any music store.

And that's it. Five simple rules, along with some ancient therapies and New Age trends, that will help you effortlessly sleep off the extra weight you've been struggling to shed. Follow the rules and suggestions faithfully. Chances are you will not only have a smile on your face when you step on the scale, you'll also have a sunnier outlook, more energy, and better focus for all the tasks and challenges that confront you each day.

1. Stick to **1** sleep schedule.
2. Starting at **2:00** p.m., eliminate all caffeine.
3. Stop alcohol **3** hours before bedtime.
4. Stop exercising **4** hours before bed.
5. Give the sun a high **5** every morning for 15 minutes.

In the chapter that follows, I will explain how to make these five rules work for you by creating your most effective sleep environment. We will explore how to choose the correct mattress, pillows, sheets, room temperature, lighting, sounds, and much more in order to help you feel drowsy and focus on rest.

7

Design the Right Environment

My patient Phoebe is an active mother of twin boys and runs marathons on many weekends. At a recent visit, she said, "Dr. Breus, I just do not have time for all this sleep hygiene and relaxation preparation. I want my body to just switch off, go to sleep, and then switch back on."

I had explained the process of sleep to Phoebe and suggested several calming techniques that touch the senses. However, she was having a difficult time making them work for her. In fact, she reported that she was beginning to feel high anxiety about the techniques because she was unable to make time for them.

So, we decided to take a step back and see if we could let her surroundings influence her senses and sleep by doing a quick bedroom makeover to create her *sleep sanctuary*. After changing the lighting, adding a simple sound (white noise) machine, and getting a more supportive mattress topper and softer pillow, Phoebe noticed such a significant difference in her ability to relax at bedtime that she actually found time to do the yoga poses starting on page 122. Since she was already in an environment promoting better rest, the relaxing poses were even more effective than we had hoped they would be!

It's important to remember that above all, *sleep is a sensory experience.* In fact, all five of your senses must be prepared for slumber in order for sleep to come easily and last all night long.

In Chapter 6, I discussed the importance of creating the right sleep routine and observing it every single day. In this chapter, I want to look at how four of the five senses—*touch, sight, sound,* and *smell*—affect your sleep. (I will discuss *taste* in Chapter 8 as I tell you what bedtime foods and snacks can help you relax and what other changes you need to make to increase your chances of getting a better night's sleep.) I have found some amazing ways to heighten these sleep senses and improve the sleep mood so that crawling into bed, closing your eyes, and drifting off to dreamland will be your greatest desire.

Do a Bedroom Check

Before you read about the sensory experience of sleep, go into your bedroom and consider the following.

1. What does your room feel like?
    - Touch your mattress. Is it firm or does it cave in to fit your body?
    - Do you wake up with lower-back pain or stiffness? How well do you sleep at a hotel?
    - Hug your pillows. Are your pillows firm but soft, or are they too flat, too hard, or too big?
    - Run your hand over your sheets. Are they smooth or rough and scratchy?

○ Squeeze your comforter or wool blanket. Is it plush, worn, or lumpy?

2. What do you see when you look around the room? How does what you see make you feel?

   ○ Do you feel tense, anxious, or relaxed?

   ○ Do you feel like you have a million things to do? Or do you feel as if this is your own private haven, just right for a mini-vacation?

   ○ Does the room have enough light? Too much light?

   ○ Is the bedroom stimulating or is there an atmosphere of relaxation?

3. What sounds do you hear in your bedroom? What sounds do you usually hear at night?

   ○ Silence? Is it too quiet?

   ○ A snoring bed partner, noisy pets, crying babies, or rambunctious kids?

   ○ Environmental sounds like horns beeping or emergency vehicles racing down the street?

   ○ The blaring television set or "You've got mail" from a family member's computer?

   ○ Your cell phone ringing?

4. Does your bedroom have a particular smell?

   ○ Is the air stale? Musty or moldy?

   ○ Does the room's scent remind you of a relaxing time in your life?

   ○ Does your bedroom smell like your pet or your favorite lotion?

When you are in your bedroom, do you want to relax, curl up, and get some much-needed rest? *Here's the ultimate question:* Is your bedroom just like any other room in the house? Is it your sleep sanctuary or is it another place to collect laundry, do work, or stress out?

If you feel no different when you walk into your bedroom, then why would your brain register anything different at bedtime, when you should feel calm, drowsy, and ready for a night's slumber?

The Sense of Touch: How Does Your Bedroom Feel?

If sleep has become your enemy, the first thing to do to design the right sleep environment is check the condition of your mattress. If you're like many people today, the mattress you sleep on is not in pristine condition. In fact, most people keep their mattresses for decades, not realizing that as people age or experience changes in fitness level, weight, or conditions such as pregnancy or back or neck pain, the mattress that was once ideal may no longer be right for them! Few people realize that the average life span of a mattress is only 7 to 8 years. This does not mean that the mattress is completely worn out after that time, but rather that your body has changed and the surface that was once supportive is no longer the right one for you or your partner.

When calculating the average life span of a mattress, we used to look at the individual components of the mattress, which can physically break down. However, it is much more important to match the materials in a mattress to changes in your body.

When to Buy a New Mattress

My friend Tina comes from a loving family that holds the value of a good night's rest in high regard. So her parents bought her a high-quality mattress when she got her first "big girl" bed (bed #1) and then another when she hit puberty (bed #2). When Tina went off to college, her dorm-room mattress was horrible, so her parents got her a mattress topper for it. When Tina moved to an apartment in her junior year in college, her mom and dad purchased another high-quality mattress (bed #3). The year she graduated, Tina got married and needed a larger mattress, because she now had a bed partner, her husband, Dave (bed #4). It wasn't long until the kids started to arrive, as did Tina's sleepless nights. By the time her second son was 3, Tina's bed had started to sag from the kids jumping on it and the many nights of ups and downs for feedings, so she replaced it (bed #5).

When Tina turned 34, her last son was born, and she and her family moved to a new home. With all the strain of lifting the three boys and moving into the home, Tina started to have lower-back pain and sought out a new mattress that would give her back better support (bed #6). Tina and Dave then went for a while with the same bed, because they were in a stable situation. No more babies were born, and both Tina and Dave stayed active with their kids, so they were trim and fit. They did not start to notice aches and pains for nearly 9 years, until Tina was 42 (bed #7).

By her late forties, Tina was experiencing early osteoarthritis and mild joint pain, which made her mattress less comfortable (leading to bed #8). With this mattress, she switched to a softer surface and slept much better. However, by age 52, she was beginning to transition into menopause, and her once-comfortable mattress felt like a furnace. She needed a surface that was cooler (bed #9), yet still supportive.

By age 60, Tina and Dave were ready to downsize. Tina wanted a bed that was supportive but had a temperature-resistant surface (bed #10). At age 68, some minor medical issues arose to bother Tina and Dave, and they both needed a bed with an adjustable base (bed #11).

At age 70, my friends have gone through 11 mattresses, getting a new one on average every 6.3 years. Let me add that they have no regrets—they consider the quality of their sleep well worth the investment!

Change your mattress based on your physical needs and life stage and on what the mattress is made of, not on the age of the mattress or what's written on the warranty. In fact, even if your physical needs do not change, you should consider investing in a new sleep surface every 7 to 8 years. To determine if you need a new mattress, here are some questions to consider.

1. How old is your mattress? Do you remember when and where you purchased it? Check your receipt file and see if you can pinpoint the mattress's age. Is it more than 8 years old? Some mattresses will have a date on the law tag.

2. How many mattresses have you purchased in your adult years? Believe it or not, the average person will need about *nine mattresses* over the course of his or her lifetime.

3. Do you wake up feeling great, or do you have pain and stiffness? If you are healthy and don't have osteoarthritis or another pain-related ailment, could the age and condition of your mattress be causing the pain?

4. Do you find that you sleep more soundly when you're away from home at a family member's house or a hotel?

DID YOU KNOW?

- If your mattress is too soft, your hips will sink in and not move, resulting in poor bloodflow and possibly strain on your upper back!
- If your mattress is too firm, you will constantly be searching for pressure relief. This will cause pain—not comfort.
- If your mattress is too soft, you will feel hotter and sweatier, and your muscles will not relax.
- If your mattress does not give you support, you cannot get proper spinal alignment at night, resulting in possible back pain and poor muscle relaxation.

MATTRESS LIFE CYCLE™ CHART

AGES	NUMBER AND TYPES OF MATTRESSES YOU'LL NEED	REASONS
0–18	**Two.** You need surfaces that adapt well to a growing body. Foam-based mattresses work well. They need to be soft because a child's body changes relatively fast. Latex and memory foam mattresses work well on both platforms and box springs.	• The needs of a growing child • The needs of a growing adolescent
19–28	**Two.** During this life stage, you need a bigger size and a more durable surface with a more supportive feel. Remember, firmness does not equal support. In many cases, a coil unit works well. For others, foam-based beds give better support.	• Size jump for marriage • Changing support needs (e.g., weight gain, kids in bed)
29–38	**Two.** A move to a new home is a good time to get a new mattress, and if lower-back pain or weight gain occurs, you need a new, more supportive surface. A coil unit may still be helpful, but start to look more closely at the memory and latex foam sleep surfaces.	• Moving to a new home • Lifestyle changes and health issues such as lower-back pain and weight gain
39–48	**One or two.** Making the move to a softer mattress may make sense at this time, depending on your medical issues. Stay away from memory foam if temperature is an issue due to night sweats or hot flashes.	• Joint degeneration, osteoarthritis, osteoporosis • Temperature sensitivity, perimenopause symptoms • Back pain, comfort problems
49–58	**One or two.** Heat retention and medical issues are the biggest concerns at this life stage. Stay away from very firm surfaces, because they increase pain. Also avoid memory foam, which heats up as you do.	• Menopause symptoms • Temperature sensitivity
59–68	**One.** Moving again to downsize also changes your bed size. You need a softer mattress for your more brittle bones, and you may develop back pain. Look for support with softness. Consider a bed with an adjustable base to help you get in and out of it.	• Medical issues • Moving to downsize household • Discomfort due to osteoarthritis, lower-back pain, or other pain conditions
69–80	**One.** At this stage you want 100 percent comfort. Get whatever feels best. Consider a bed with an adjustable base.	• Making final major purchases • New medical issues

Pick Mattress Pads, Covers, and Protectors

If you have purchased a new mattress or topper, then you need to protect your investment. Look for mattress pads and covers that will protect against liquid spills, urine, and blood, as well as dust mites and other allergens.

Types of Pads, Covers, and Protectors

Mattress pads are primarily used for adding a thin extra layer of comfort while also protecting the surface from stains and spills. These will interfere with the way memory foam works. Mattress protectors are best if incontinence or kids in the bed are possibilities.

There are different types of pads, covers, and protectors that can encase mattresses, box springs, and pillows. These protectors are usually made of vinyl, cotton, or newer materials that allow for ventilation while still maintaining a barrier between liquids and your mattress.

The Best Mattress Protector Features

When selecting the best mattress cover or protector, look for the following.

- A waterproof (not water-resistant) material that allows for proper ventilation while keeping dust mites from finding a breeding ground in your mattress. Vinyl does not breathe well.
- It should fully enclose your mattress. The zipper or hook-and-loop (i.e., Velcro) seal is one of the most important features, because it can keep everything away from the mattress. Make sure the seal is not broken.
  - The zipper should be coated to prevent rust.
  - There should be an extra flap of fabric that covers the zipper itself as well as the seam.

Select your mattress protector carefully, because many lower-end products will not have all the features you need.

Pick the Perfect Pillow

Having a perfect bedroom involves more than getting a good mattress. Pillows are serious sleep products that have a big impact on both your sleep and your overall health. But how much do you really know about pillows? When you go to a popular bed or linens store and see a gigantic pillow wall, how do you select the best pillow for you? As a *Sleep Doctor,* I believe that you should have pillow choices—like your own private pillow menu—in order to get the best quality of sleep each night.

The main purpose of a pillow is to align the cervical spine (the part in your neck) so there is no flexion (bend) or tension (muscle tightness) in the neck during sleep. If a pillow is too plump (i.e., pushes the chin into the chest for back sleepers or lifts the head toward the ceiling for side sleepers), then it is not doing a proper job. Look at the drawings below and see if your current pillow fits into the Just Right category. Go ahead and ask your bed partner or a close friend to look at your head and neck when you are in your starting sleep position. Ask him or her if there is alignment. If there isn't, you need to consider buying a new pillow.

CHOOSE THE RIGHT PILLOW FOR THE BEST SLEEP

FOR BACK SLEEPERS

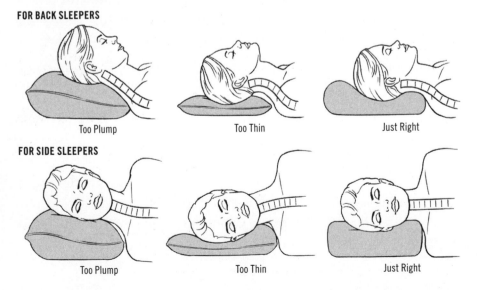

| Too Plump | Too Thin | Just Right |

FOR SIDE SLEEPERS

| Too Plump | Too Thin | Just Right |

The second purpose of a pillow is to provide comfort—it needs to feel good! This requires getting the right pillow size, shape, and fill for your sleep position. To find the right pillow, you only need to answer these three simple questions.

1. Do you like your pillow to feel solid (all one piece) or soft and squishy (stuffing)?
2. What position do you start sleeping in? On your back, side, or stomach?
3. Do you have any neck or back pain?

Now follow the *Pic-a-Pillow Chart* to find your best pillow.

PIC-A-PILLOW CHART

Note: *If you are experiencing neck pain, confirm these pillow shapes and sizes with your doctor!*

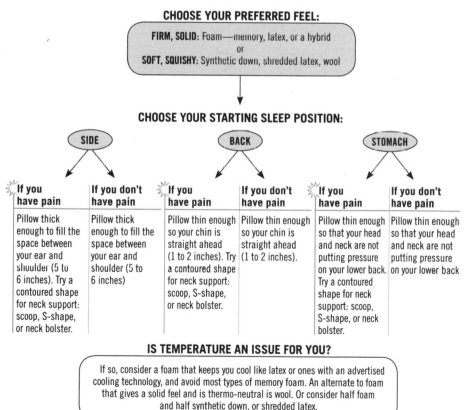

CHOOSE YOUR PREFERRED FEEL:

FIRM, SOLID: Foam—memory, latex, or a hybrid
or
SOFT, SQUISHY: Synthetic down, shredded latex, wool

CHOOSE YOUR STARTING SLEEP POSITION:

SIDE · BACK · STOMACH

If you have pain	If you don't have pain	If you have pain	If you don't have pain	If you have pain	If you don't have pain
Pillow thick enough to fill the space between your ear and shoulder (5 to 6 inches). Try a contoured shape for neck support: scoop, S-shape, or neck bolster.	Pillow thick enough to fill the space between your ear and shoulder (5 to 6 inches)	Pillow thin enough so your chin is straight ahead (1 to 2 inches). Try a contoured shape for neck support: scoop, S-shape, or neck bolster.	Pillow thin enough so your chin is straight ahead (1 to 2 inches).	Pillow thin enough so that your head and neck are not putting pressure on your lower back. Try a contoured shape for neck support: scoop, S-shape, or neck bolster.	Pillow thin enough so that your head and neck are not putting pressure on your lower back

IS TEMPERATURE AN ISSUE FOR YOU?

If so, consider a foam that keeps you cool like latex or ones with an advertised cooling technology, and avoid most types of memory foam. An alternate to foam that gives a solid feel and is thermo-neutral is wool. Or consider half foam and half synthetic down, or shredded latex.

Select the Best Comforter, Spread, or Duvet

Just as the right mattress can help sleep issues disappear, so too can your comforter, spread, and duvet have a huge impact on your sleep. A comforter is much like a blanket and is used on top of the top sheet or a light blanket. The comforter is built for warmth, and it's primarily used in the colder months. A decorative spread may be lightweight and is used to cover the sheets when the bed is not being used. A duvet (French for "down") can be filled with down, feathers, or a combination of the two and is generally inserted into a fabric cover. Duvets are sometimes used in place of a top sheet. All of these products will help maintain temperature and control humidity, both of which affect your sleep.

Choose the Best Materials

Wool fabrics breathe well and are great insulators. The good ventilation you get with wool helps to diminish temperature swings that can disrupt your sleep. Wool is cool in the summer and warm in the winter, and doesn't weigh as much as some down- or fiber-filled comforters. I use a wool comforter year-round.

Down feels luxurious and comforting. When you sleep surrounded by down, pressure points on the body are relieved. Down feathers are like natural springs, so some women report a reduction in pain and better sleep. Down is insulating and is a good choice for those who sleep in a cooler environment, because it keeps the temperature more comfortable and less prone to fluctuation.

Polyester is best used during winter months, because it has a tendency to retain heat and doesn't breathe as well. Because of the poor ventilation, the air temperature under your covers will rise with your body temperature. When your body cools for sleep, the environment under the covers will still feel toasty! A polyester comforter may be fine for a guest bed, but it's not really something you will want on your bed every night unless the temperature in your bedroom is brutally cold.

Silk comforters today are priced similarly to down comforters. Silk is naturally hypoallergenic and does not require the application of chemicals during the manufacturing process. For women with allergies to down, silk is a great alternative, because sneezing and nasal congestion can have a detrimental effect on sleep.

Pick the Best Features

- **Hypoallergenic**—Most natural fibers and fills can have allergens, so beware of those that claim otherwise. Nasal congestion will increase snoring, so select synthetic materials that are labeled hypoallergenic for better breathing and more peaceful sleep.
- **Washable**—Being able to wash a comforter or duvet is an important feature, especially if you use it without a top sheet. Your sweat and skin oils will wick into the fabric unless you have it in a cover or encasement that is removable, which I recommend.
- **Stitching**—Quilting allows the fill to stay consistently distributed inside the cover.
- **Flame-retardant**—Using less-flammable bedclothes is a good idea, but remember that flame-retardant does not mean fireproof.

Select Sensual Sheets

I never really thought about sheets until my wife and I were engaged. Before the wedding, we were at a department store registering our gift choices with the price gun. When we got to the bedding section, my soon-to-be wife grabbed the gun and said, "This one is all me!" I had never really had an appreciation of what a difference really good sheets make. Since then, I have learned just how much more comfortable great sheets can feel.

There are several things to think about when selecting sheets for great sleep. Sizing and fit both play roles. You want a sheet that fits snugly so when you and your partner move around, you won't disturb each other's sleep. Sheets that bunch or gather can get caught up in someone's legs and tug at the other person.

Size. It is a good idea to measure your mattress and have these measurements with you when you go shopping. Of particular importance is the pocket depth—the actual measurement from the bottom edge of the mattress to the top. If you have a pillow top mattress or top your mattress with a memory foam pad or another liner, you may need to buy sheets with deeper pockets to accommodate it, even if your mattress is of a standard size.

- **Standard pocket size—**7 to 9 inches (18 to 23 centimeters)
- **Deep pocket size—**10 to 15 inches (25 to 38 centimeters)
- **Extra-deep pocket size—**15 to 22 inches (38 to 56 centimeters)

Fit. All fitted sheets are not created equal! The determining factor in suitability (besides the material, which is discussed in the next section) is the elastic on it. Here are some typical options you can find.

- Elastic is only at the corners (with these, sheets can come off in the middle of the night).
- Elastic runs down both sides.
- Elastic goes all the way around to keep the sheets in place.

Now, How Does It Feel?

The material your sheets are made of, including its weave, fit, and thread count, is an important aspect of the textile that spends more time touching your skin than any other fabric. Sheets confer comfort, and the more comfortable you feel in bed, the faster you will fall asleep . . . and stay asleep.

The feel of your sheets can help you relax. Your level of comfort in bed is directly related to the ease of going to sleep. Consider the following to find the greatest comfort in sheets.

Thread count. Thread count (also called "threads per inch") is the number of threads per square inch of material. This number includes the threads running in both directions, vertically and horizontally. As a general rule, standard cotton sheets' thread counts are about 150, and sheets of medium quality have thread counts of about 180. Material having a count of more than 200 is called "percale." The higher the thread count, the longer lasting and more luxurious the sheet or fabric.

Types. There are so many types of textiles used to make bedding. Here, your personal preference often dictates the best choice, unless heat and moisture are issues when you sleep. Choose from the following:

- **Muslin**—Muslin can feel scratchy due to its thread count of 128 to 140. This cotton fabric is often used in kids' novelty or printed sheets.

- **Combed cotton**—Combing cotton removes the short fibers, making the fabric smoother.

- **Pima cotton**—This longer cotton fiber is grown primarily in the American Southwest. Supima is even longer, and both tend to have thread counts of 200 to 300.

- **Egyptian cotton**—This cotton is grown only along the Egyptian section of the Nile River and is considered the best, since the fabric has very long fibers that make thinner thread. Its thread count is high, usually 200 or more.

- **Jersey**—This is a plain knit fabric.

- **Linen**—Linen is a fiber made from flax, but it is rarely used for bedding anymore because it wrinkles easily and requires ironing for comfortable sleep.

- **Modal**—Modal is a cellulose fiber similar to rayon.
- **Percale**—A cotton or cotton-polyester plain-weave fabric, percale has equal or similar vertical and horizontal thread counts.
- **Plain weave**—The simplest weave structure, fabric made this way has single vertical and horizontal threads woven under and over.
- **Polyester**—This synthetic fiber can sleep very hot!
- **Sateen**—Sateen is a smooth, fairly glossy cotton fabric made by weaving horizontal threads over four or more vertical threads. The textile used is often cotton.
- **Satin**—This fabric is woven in the same way as sateen but with silk, nylon, or polyester threads.
- **Silk**—This organic material is incredibly soft but requires dry cleaning.
- **Bamboo**—This is one of the newest fabrics being marketed in the bedding world, and it is thought to have natural cooling properties.

For the Best Sheets, Consider This
- Select pima or Egyptian cotton or sateen
- Look for a 350 thread count
- Opt for lighter colors
- Get a fitted sheet with a full elastic band. Throw in a bamboo set for a great feel!

Sight: Light Is Your Biological Reset Button

Your brain uses the sense of sight to interpret light, which influences your ability to fall asleep more than any other factor. There has been a great deal of research on the effects of light on sleep. As noted in Chapter 6, sleep specialists use light therapy to help people fall asleep and stay asleep at the right times for their schedules, but it is equally important to ensure that you don't expose your eyes to light at the *wrong* times. Here are some of the lighting considerations you should review when evaluating your sleep environment.

- **Room lighting—**The room lights need to be dimmed to less than 200 watts total from all light sources 1 hour before the lights are turned off for sleep. Total bedroom wattage is important. High wattage may prevent the production of melatonin, the hormone that makes you feel sleepy at night.
- **Room color—**Choose flat finish paint for your bedroom. Use no more than three colors, and make sure the colors represent tranquillity to you. A vibrantly colored room may unconsciously make you think of something disturbing that could prevent sleep or affect your dreams.
- **Book light—**Get a book light that is battery operated, casts light on both pages, and is easy to use.
- **Sleep mask—**The sleep mask (also called an eye mask) you select should block light completely but be comfortable all night long. These are great sleep aids, particularly when traveling by airplane or car.
- **Blackout curtains—**These curtains should block 99 percent of light and completely cover the entire window and casing. Remember, a dark room is more conducive to falling asleep.

Room Lighting

Clearly the size of the bedroom and the room lighting type (natural and/or artificial) will have a huge impact on your overall experience of your sleep environment. One of my first recommendations for any bedroom is to *install a dimmer switch.* Remember, light prevents the initiation of sleep because it compromises the body's ability to produce melatonin.

In addition, consider using bedside table lamps as opposed to track lighting or recessed "cans" in the ceiling. I prefer nonhalogen 45-watt "natural light" bulbs in bedside lamps. If you do not want a low-wattage bulb, get a dimmer cord or a screw-in bulb switch that gives any lamp dimmer capability. (These are called *touch dimmers* and are available at most hardware stores.)

Here are some general guidelines for bedroom lighting.

- **Dimmer is better**—Because our brains are designed to slow down when the sun goes down, make your bedroom feel like dusk 1 hour before bedtime.
- **Natural light**—Many of the newer lightbulbs have a natural light option that filters out many of the brighter light wavelengths. If you have a skylight, keep it uncovered at night and allow the natural light of the evening to flow in. This option can also make for nice stargazing, which can be relaxing.
- **Overhead fan lighting**—If you have an overhead fan with a light kit, use this as the main source of light. Make sure the bulbs are about 45 watts, which provides enough light to see but not enough to disrupt your melatonin production, letting you fall asleep easily.

Add Night-Lights

You should be able to get up in the middle of the night without having to turn on an overhead light. If you do turn on a light, your brain will think morning has come and will stop producing melatonin. To avoid this, install night-lights in your hallways and bathroom, making sure they are small, ambient lights—not too bright. I have seen some small spotlight types or directional lights that point toward the floor, and these should be avoided.

Types of Night-Lights

- **Motion-sensor night-lights—**These night-lights are great for both energy savings and functionality. They will not keep you up at night, but should you need to move about, they will illuminate your path without telling your brain that daybreak has arrived. Do consider the range of the sensor when placing your night-lights; you do not want to get out of bed and have to walk all the way across the room before the light goes on. A word of caution: Pets love to play with these once they figure them out!

- **Decorative night-lights—**While you want the night-light to be functional, you also want it to be discreet. Make sure that the night-light blends well with the decor, if possible.

- **Blue-light night-lights—**These are night-lights that use a special blue-light wavelength that will not halt the production of melatonin.

Television at Night

Like daylight, televisions (and computer screens) emit bright light that to your brain simulates being out in the sunlight, inhibiting this production of melatonin and disrupting your sleep rhythms. For this reason, I recommend turning off the TV in the bedroom. However, many people like to fall asleep to the TV. If you are one of those people, make sure you set your TV sleep timer so the set will turn itself off soon after you fall asleep. That way the light from the TV won't tell your brain it's time to wake up.

You might also consider purchasing a TV or computer screen filter, which filters out the light that prevents melatonin from being produced. This product enables you to watch TV or check your e-mail and still be able to fall asleep when you are ready.

THE LOWDOWN ON BOOK LIGHTS

Reading at night is a great way to wind down and relax. However, I recommend that people use a book light rather than a bedside table lamp when reading in bed. Choose one that is small, compact, lightweight, and battery operated or rechargeable and features multiple light sources to avoid eyestrain. Here are some widely available options.

Clip-on with flexible neck. These are ideal because you can adjust the light source.

Clip-on with double neck. There are two light sources with these, one for each page of an open book.

Around the neck. This one sits on your chest and has two light sources.

On the ear. This spotlight fits over your ear like a hands-free device for your cell phone.

On the page. One book light is a small piece of Plexiglas that sits on the book page itself. The light source shoots across the entire sheet, causing the whole page to light up. These book lights come in paperback and hardcover sizes, and the light doubles as a bookmark.

Paint Your Room Peaceful

For years I have heard designers say that color influences their clients' moods and emotions. Recently, I reviewed a meta-analysis that concluded that we do indeed have emotional responses to particular colors. These responses are culturally learned associations, suggesting that our choices of colors are influenced by our experiences with these colors and their significance to our cultures and lives. For example, if you want your bedroom to feel open and airy, you will want contrasting colors that make you feel tranquil and calm. If a wooded area seems peaceful to you, consider using two different shades of deep green to create the ambience of a forest.

Color associations to consider when choosing bedroom colors:

- **Cream or white**—Softness and purity (like angels)
- **Purple or lavender**—Royalty and tranquillity (represented in nature by the flowers of the herbs lavender and periwinkle)
- **Green**—Growth, Mother Earth, calm
- **Brown (earth tones)**—Nature, autumn, peacefulness
- **Blue**—Ocean, sky

Consider Wearing an Eyeshade or Sleep Mask

Eyeshades and sleep masks (also called eye masks) are healthy components of your overall sleep environment. We know that light decreases the production of melatonin, so the less light you see at night, the better you will sleep. If you live near a streetlight, have a bed partner who is afraid of the dark, or like sleeping with the window open, then an eyeshade or sleep mask can be the perfect solution.

You want it to be made of a material that is durable, washable, breathable, and attractive. Washability is very important because you sweat when you sleep, plus your skin has oils that rub off onto fabrics.

Your sleep mask should have good straps that will hold it in place comfortably throughout the night. Those with single elastic straps are the least expensive, but they also rarely stay in place. Sleep masks with more than one strap tend to have more support and stay put.

Consider Installing Blackout Curtains

Blackout curtains are important if you are light sensitive and cannot sleep with a sleep mask. The three main functions of blackout curtains are:

- **To block out light**—Depending upon the materials and construction, you may get 99 to 100 percent blockage.

- **To block out exterior noise**—Blackout curtains are a good adjunct to a sound-masking machine (page 154), because they can block up to 40 percent of external noise.
- **An added bonus: to save energy**—Ten to 25 percent of thermal energy loss goes out through the windows.

There are two basic types of blackout curtains.

- **Curtains with a backing**—The backing can be a plastic sheet or another textile that has a tightly woven fabric.
- **Sandwich-type curtains**—This type has a material such as plastic or a tightly woven textile sandwiched between two other fabrics.

Here are the features you will want to evaluate when purchasing blackout curtains.

- **Are they wide enough?** For larger windows, custom curtains may be needed, since your curtain is only as good as the area it covers. If there is the smallest space between the panels or between your curtains and the window frame, light will wake you up!
- **Do the panels attach in some way?** Some curtains have a hook-and-loop strip that attaches the panels to one another; others have small snaps. Such closures may not be necessary if your curtains hang correctly. Note that if you have curtains you love but find a gap that admits light into the room, you can try using a kitchen clip to keep them closed.

Sound: Your Inner Sleep Security System

It should come as no surprise that you can still hear external sounds while you are sleeping. Parents awaken to a baby's cry, or the sound of an intruder may wake you. Perhaps the disruptive sound that's keeping you awake is your partner's snoring or the sounds made by your pet at the foot of your bed. When there is a noise in the sleep laboratory, we can observe the effect on the patient's brain waves, even if the noise does not awaken the patient.

Interestingly, the human ear is not the only anatomical part of the body that perceives sound. Only about 35 percent of what we hear is based on sound waves going into the ear canal. The rest is picked up as vibrations bouncing off the bones surrounding the ear. That is why earplugs are one of the least effective methods blocking noise during sleep. Also, the quieter the bedroom, the more sensitive your hearing becomes. Some of my patients report that when they travel, they find the new environment "too quiet for sleep." This is why a multifaceted approach to sound and sleep may be needed. Before we begin, here is a list of the most important recommendations for each potential remedy.

- **Earplugs**—Comfort is key, especially for side sleepers. Make sure your plugs have a noise reduction rating of 32 decibels or below so you can still hear a smoke alarm or a child in distress.
- **White noise or sound machines**—These machines need to produce a sound that has no particular meaning or association for you (other than relaxation). Some machines can actually increase the complexity of the sound they emit as new sounds appear throughout the night.
- **Alarm clocks**—Feature choice is the most important factor, and this is individual to each sleeper.

End Nighttime Noise with Earplugs

There are three types of earplugs used to reduce nighttime noise.

- **Foam earplugs**—These are usually made of memory foam, which is compressed and then placed in the ear canal, where the foam expands to block sound waves.

- **Silicone earplugs**—These are rolled into a tiny ball and then carefully molded to fit over the external part of the ear canal to give the wearer a snug fit.
- **Flanged earplugs**—These are the custom-molded types that most musicians use.

Earplugs do not all fit the same. Try on the earplugs while lying down, because the pressure on the ear from the head and the pillow may cause a significant reduction in comfort. Also, just tilting the head back or to the side causes major anatomical changes in the ear canal, which can cause the plug to loosen. To get a complete seal, you have to wait about 20 seconds for the earplug to expand fully inside the ear canal.

Do choose plugs that are comfortable. If you cannot stand wearing them, you will remove them at night, maybe even while you are asleep. Plugs are noise reduction rated. This number corresponds to the number of decibels that will be blocked. A noise level rating of about 32 decibels is the highest you want. It will block about a third of the noise in the environment but still allow you to hear emergency situations.

Plugs should be thrown away (if foam) or washed (if silicone or flanged) to avoid earwax buildup and uncleanliness.

Consider Sound Machines

As I mentioned with respect to earplugs, the quieter the environment is, the more sensitive your hearing becomes, with the result that you might hear things that you would not in a louder environment.

Sound masking is adding a soothing natural or artificial sound to cover other, more distracting sounds. **White noise** is produced by combining the sounds of all the different frequencies. It's thought that sound machines improve sleep in the following ways.

- Allowing the person to fall asleep faster by masking distracting noises

- Allowing the person to be awakened fewer times by unwanted noises

The Types of Sound Machines

Most sound machines have speaker systems, are self-contained units, and produce reasonably good-quality sound. There are a few differentiating features.

White noise only. A basic, no-frills white noise generator is better than a fan or air conditioner and works best for some women.

Mixed sounds. This type of sound machine has options for white noise plus nature sounds or a complex set of layered sounds.

Multifunction. This type includes a sound machine plus an alarm clock and radio. They may not be as effective for sleep, given some of the additional features. See my discussion of alarm clocks on page 156.

Key Features to Think About

Sound quality. Pay attention to the sound quality and speakers (if included). Some machines have multiple speakers that are detachable, and some have built-in tweeters, subwoofers, and all the other things you pay attention to in a nice stereo system. But you do not need to be an audiophile to find a good white noise machine. It is unlikely that top-of-the-line speakers will significantly improve the average person's ability to fall or stay asleep.

Masking ability. Can the machine mask snoring, road noise, a barking dog?

Types of sounds. Having different types of sounds may be better than the standard white noise. Some machines use nature sounds, including one with upwards of 20 sounds. I even saw one with 120 soundscape possibilities! Some of the options include:

- Water-based sounds, such as ocean surf, a babbling brook, a rainstorm, or a waterfall

- Animal-based sounds, including crickets on a summer night and a human heartbeat
- Environmental noises like a faraway train, city street noise, a log burning in a fireplace, a rain forest, or a thunderstorm
- Meditation- or relaxation-promoting sounds such as instrumental music or a person's voice guiding you through a meditation
- White noise, which is a single meaningless sound similar to static on the radio

Volume. Can you control the volume? There are now sound machines that will not only produce sound at a constant volume, but also raise and lower the volume depending upon the current environmental sounds (think snoring that changes in volume!).

Portability. Is the machine small enough to take with you on a trip and to fit easily on your nightstand?

Timer. A timer can shut off the machine after a certain length of time, such as 15, 30, 45, or 60 minutes. There are also some with nap timers.

Intelligent machines. These machines have sensors that determine what sounds are audible in the room and then produce an appropriate masking sound.

Now, Wake Up . . . and Find the Best Alarm Clock

If your sleep-wake rhythm is aligned correctly and you get up at the same time each day, then you shouldn't need to use an alarm clock. But most people need them to function and to ensure that they get where they need to go in a timely fashion—or just as a backup in case their internal clocks go on the fritz. When you are looking for an alarm clock, ask yourself these questions.

How do you prefer to be awakened? (No, this is not a trick question!)

- By sound
- By light

- By vibration
- By a combination

Who needs to be awakened by this alarm?

- You
- Your bed partner
- Only one bed partner

Are there any special considerations to keep in mind for you or your bed partner?

- Deep sleeper
- Very difficult to wake up
- Sensitive to light
- Sensitive to sound

Digital. Digital alarm clocks display the numbers in a variety of colors. Some let you turn the light down or even off. I saw one digital alarm clock with a motion sensor that turns the clock light on when you wave your hand in front of it. Now, that's pretty cool!

Analog. This is the classic face-with-hands model. Most, if not all, analog clocks have illuminated hands these days.

Wake-up feature options give you the ability to:

- Be awakened by a preset alarm tone
- Be awakened by a radio station, weather sounds, a CD, or nature sounds
- Be awakened by a vibrating disk placed inside your pillow or under your mattress
- Be awakened by a graduating light (yes, your room gets brighter over time)

- Be awakened by aromatherapy scents ranging from peppermint to coffee and even bacon!
- Set dual alarms
  - For two different people
  - For weekends versus weekdays

Cope with the Sounds of Snoring

Snoring is the number one reason why so many people across the country seek out sleep doctors. They cannot get adequate rest when they're sleeping next to a freight train. One patient told me that her husband's snoring was so loud that she made him sleep in the car in the garage just so she could get some peace and quiet. While this was an extreme situation, it is not uncommon to have one partner banished from the couple's bedroom because of snoring.

Approximately 90 million American adults snore, and of those individuals, 37 million snore on a regular basis.[1] Snoring is a problem among all age groups and both genders, but up to a certain age, more men snore than women. After menopause, women are just as likely to snore as men. Chronic snoring is associated with an increased incidence of heart disease and stroke because it leads to high blood pressure. Up to 20 percent of those who snore have sleep apnea.

The Science of Snoring

While you sleep, your respiratory system is hard at work. The muscles at the back of your throat relax while your diaphragm—the large muscle that lies below your lungs and makes them expand and deflate—continues its pumping action. The excessive relaxation of the muscles in the mouth and throat results in a narrowing of the trachea, diminishing airflow. The soft palate and uvula (that fleshy structure that hangs down from your soft palate) at the back of your throat may shake, flop back and forth, or vibrate, causing the annoying noises we call snoring. When the throat is obstructed for even just a few seconds, a temporary cessation of breathing known as apnea happens. When apneas last long enough—they can be up to a couple of minutes long—you may experience a drop in your blood oxygen level. Left untreated, apnea can lead to a host of other serious problems.[2]

Sleeping with a Noisy Bed Partner

A 2001 survey by the National Sleep Foundation found that more than 1 in 10 married couples are sleeping in separate beds. Because we spend about a third of our married lives in bed sleeping with our partners, it is very important to make sure that your sleep styles are compatible so you can both get a restful night's sleep. If you are a snorer who's driven away a sleep partner, here are steps you can take to control your snoring and increase the quality and quantity of your sleep.

- Lose weight if you are overweight. A 5 percent drop in weight can make a significant difference in snoring.
- Seek medical treatment for allergies or respiratory problems that cause snoring.
- Ask your doctor to check for upper airway obstructions such as enlarged tonsils or adenoids, polyps, or a deviated nasal septum.
- Avoid sleeping on your back.
- Avoid heavy meals before bedtime.
- Some medications, such as antihistamines, sleeping pills, and tranquilizers, can add to a snoring problem. Talk to your doctor if you are taking any of these medications to see if there are alternative drugs that might help your situation.
- If you smoke cigarettes, stop.
- Avoid drinking alcohol close to bedtime.
- If your snorer has any congestion, ask your doctor about a nasal decongestant.
- Put a pillow between you and your snoring partner. Remember, snoring is a soundwave that can be blocked.

Manage Noisy Pets

Interestingly, a 2001 survey by the Mayo Clinic Sleep Disorders Center revealed that 53 percent of people who slept with their pets claimed the animals disturbed their sleep.[3] My professional experience also shows that pet owners who allow pets into their beds have a higher percentage of sleep problems than those who don't.

In addition to disturbed sleep due to pet-related allergies, pet owners may also lose sleep because animals don't have the same sleep-wake cycle that we do. (Maybe we are also disturbing our pets' sleep each night!) Cats can be active in the late-night and early morning hours and thus might disrupt these hours of your sleep. Even a dog in the bed can disrupt the owner with all the scratching, sniffing, snoring, and moving around. A recent study found that some pets may carry disease or other pests, like fleas or bedbugs.

In addition, cats' claws can catch on bedclothes, ripping them and ruining your investment. If you do let your cat sleep with you, avoid snags by trimming his or her nails regularly or gluing those plastic covers over the claws.

Survival Strategies for Kids and Sleep

In my clinical experience, having children is a key factor in sleep disturbances for women. I say this because no matter what her age, almost every mom I treat says, "Once I had kids, I never slept the same again."

Sure, some moms get great sleep! But when speaking honestly, most moms agree that with kids come sleep issues. Here are some tips for helping kids get their sleep—so you can get yours.

Try a Kid Power-Down Hour. For kids, the time before bed can be quite different than it is for adults. In many cases with a working parent, the parent may not get home until later (usually within an hour of the child's bedtime). This can result in the child's missing his or her scheduled bedtime. Especially with boys and their fathers, I often see

! SLEEP ALERT Sleep apnea is of growing concern to pediatricians today. Check out the information on sleep apnea (page 34) and see if your child might have the symptoms. Talk to a pediatric sleep specialist for diagnosis and treatment.

wrestling and physical play before bed. Though fun, this can have the opposite effect of making a child sleepy.

In addition, the timing of dinner can be a significant factor in the child's getting the right amount of sleep at the right time. Serve dinner 2 hours before bedtime. This will allow time for digestion and help avoid stomachaches.

Plan bedtimes according to the following:

BEDTIMES FOR KIDS BASED ON A 7 A.M. WAKE-UP TIME

AGE	BEDTIME
1 year	8 p.m. and 2 daytime naps for about 90 min.
1–2 years	8 p.m. and 2 daytime naps for about 60 min.
2–3 years	8 p.m. and 1 daytime nap for about 60 min.
3–5 years	7:30 p.m.
5–8 years	8 p.m.
8–11 years	9 p.m.
11–14 years	9:30 p.m.
14–16 years	10 p.m.
16+ years	10:30 p.m.

Next, use the *Kid Power-Down Hour* to stack the deck for a good night's rest.

- **First 20 minutes**—All electronics must be turned off. During this time, your child or teen can finish up homework, get clothes together for school, and set his or her schedules for the week.

- **Second 20 minutes**—The child or teen should do any personal hygiene needed, such as taking a warm bath or shower, brushing the teeth, washing the face, and applying any necessary creams and gels.

- **Final 20 minutes**—Read a bedtime story to younger children. Older children and teens can read quietly in their bedrooms.

The key to the entire process is to stick to a regular schedule and keep the activities before bed sleep friendly.

CONGESTED AND CAN'T SLEEP?

While incredibly simple, a sinus wash using a saline solution is an effective method of reducing congestion. Neti pots have a small, spouted pitcher used to introduce warm water into the sinus cavity, been around for centuries and originally come from the ayurvedic/yoga medical tradition (page 121). You can also use a plastic squirt bottle or even a cupped hand to "snort" the saline solution.

To use a neti pot, fill the base of the pot with 8 ounces of warm (not hot) water and $\frac{1}{2}$ teaspoon of noniodized salt. Then, tilting your head to the side over the sink, pour the solution into one nostril and let it drain out the other while breathing through your mouth. Exhale sharply through your nose to clear mucus from the nostril. Then refill the pot and do the same on the other side. Blow your nose thoroughly to further clear the nasal passages when you're finished.

At first, pouring saline solution through your nose may feel strange. But you will get used to the feeling of salt water in your nose and possibly a little dripping down the back of your throat. Once the congestion has been reduced, regular saline irrigation three times per week is usually enough to clear out the sinuses.

The Sweet Smell of Sleep: Aromatherapy, Air Quality, and Humidity

Smell is one of the least understood of the five senses, yet it is a powerful sense in its own right. When a scent goes into your nose, it crosses the olfactory membrane and stimulates the olfactory nerve. This nerve communicates directly with an area in the brain called the limbic system, where memory, hunger, sexual response, and emotion are evoked. Here are some ways you can harness this powerful sensory response to aid in your quest for better sleep.

- **Air purifiers**—Clean air can improve your ability to breathe, which will positively affect your sleep. An air filter is a great way to improve air quality, but some are pretty complicated.
- **Humidity**—The amount of moisture in the air affects how easily you breathe during sleep. There are many different humidifiers on the market, so look for one that is adequate for your bedroom size.

Aromatherapy

While aromatherapy is really more for relaxation than for sleep, the pleasurable scents are still effective. Certain scents are more effective than others, and you do not need to perfume your entire room to get a drowsy effect. You may have experienced a certain fragrance brightening your mood or even relaxing you when you were stressed. For instance, the smells of lavender and spiced apples are both thought to activate alpha wave activity at the back of the brain, which leads to relaxation. Jasmine and lemon increase beta wave activity in the front of the brain, which is associated with alertness.

Lavender in particular has been shown in some studies to help with sleep by increasing the percentage of deep sleep for both men and women.[4] Additionally, those who use lavender for sleep report having more vigor (energy) in the morning.[5] On the flip side, stay away from peppermint and other minty scents in the evening. These have been shown to have an alerting effect rather than a sedating one.

There are numerous methods for using aromatherapy, from scented drawer liners to elaborate vaporizer machines that release a mist of fragrance by gently heating dried herbs or potpourri. Choose the one that feels most comfortable and relaxing to you.

Massage oil. My favorite vehicle for aromatherapy is massage oil. To the scents' sedative properties, you add the soothing qualities of the massage itself.

Baths. My second-favorite way to use natural aromatherapy is in bathwater. Taking a warm bath can also help improve sleep by causing an increase in core body temperature, which will then lead to melatonin production when the body cools.

Candles. This is my least-favorite way to apply aromatherapy because fire and sleep do not mix! That said, there are some new candles that go out if they are tipped over and may be a safer alternative.

Plug-ins. These scented devices work well and usually are not fire hazards. However, finding good-quality essential oils to refill these mass-produced devices may be difficult.

Pillow sachet. This method can make the scent more available to the user while not bothering the bed partner. However, some women report that their hair retains the smell in the morning.

Pillow spray. This is an excellent application method, but patients again complain that their hair smells the next day. (Also watch out if you find out overnight that you are allergic to the scent—you'll need to wash your hair to remove the fragrance.)

Diffuser. This is one of the most popular methods for using aromatherapy. A diffuser is an electric or metal lamp ring with a channel for holding oil that you place on top of a lightbulb to warm.

Consider the Best Oils for Sleep

Essential oils are the purest form of fragrance available and often are found only at specialty stores or natural food stores. They can be quite expensive, but the purity is worth the price. If you make your own pillow spray from pure essential oil, you will save money and get an incredible scent.

- Lavender has the most data on effectiveness and is the scent that most people associate with sleep.
- Chamomile is an herb used for tea, but it can also have a relaxing effect when used for aromatherapy.
- Ylang-ylang is an herb that has been shown in some studies to promote relaxation and better sleep.

Discover More about Air Quality, Humidity, and Your Sleep

One of the aspects we may overlook with respect to our sleep environment is the air we breathe. Air quality and humidity have key effects on our sleep. About 90 percent of the time we spend at home is indoors, so air quality can be an unrecognized sleep stealer. Irritating or toxic substances in the air can increase the risk of upper respiratory infections and allergy attacks—conditions that can keep you awake all night long. So, what contributes to poor air quality?

- Cigarette smoke
- Dust
- Gases and smoke from a furnace, stove, or water heater
- Pet dander
- Pollen
- Poor ventilation

To keep the air inside your home as irritant free and fresh as possible, try to open your windows at least once a week and get air flowing through the rooms. If the weather or your location makes this difficult, you should investigate buying an air filter to extract potential irritants and pollutants from the air circulating through your home. Change your air filters once a month and get outside as often as you can.

About Air Filters and Purifiers

Air filters are designed to remove particulates (dust, pollen, molds, and bacteria) from the air. There are room filters sold as stand-alone units called air purifiers and entire-house filters that are placed inside your heating, ventilation, and air-conditioning unit. When you are considering buying an air filter, you will want to think about several factors.

- What types of particles are you trying to get rid of?
- Does the filter meet high-efficiency particulate air (HEPA) filter standards? Check to see if your HVAC unit can handle this type of very fine filtration.
- What is the clean air delivery rate of the filter?
- Is changing the filters easy?
- If it's a room unit, how much noise does it make?

To select the proper air filter, you need to know the size of the particles you are trying to filter out of your air. Allergens are measured in microns (to give you a point of reference, a human hair is about 70 microns thick). The body's normal defense (tiny hairs in your nose, sinuses, and windpipe) is designed to filter out particles larger than about 3 to 5 microns, but clearly this does not get them all.

The good news here is that a HEPA filter appears to filter out particles down to about 0.3 microns. The bad news is that if your furnace and HVAC system are not designed for a HEPA filter, the fineness of the filter can put a strain on the system, use more energy, and cause the system to wear out faster. Look at your home owner's manual or on the side of your HVAC unit to see if the system can handle a HEPA filter. To filter out tobacco smoke, you will need a gas air purifier.

There are many ways that your sleep environment can help you get a better night's rest. You should now have a good idea of how you can engage your senses of touch, sight, sound, and smell to enhance your sleep experience.

But what about taste? Did you know that the food you eat can have an impact on your sleep (or lack of sleep)? In the next chapter, I will give you information on foods that can calm you down, make you feel drowsy, and allow you to get more sleep so you can lose weight and feel great.

8

Eat Right to Sleep Tight

Chances are that you bought this book because you need to lose some weight. So why am I suggesting that you eat to lose weight? Because eating the right foods—and avoiding the wrong ones—*will make it easier for you to fall asleep and stay asleep.* And sleeping longer will not only help you to lose weight, but also, according to a new study published in the *Annals of Internal Medicine,* make you feel *less hungry* while you're awake.[1]

When the dieters in this particular study got up to 8.5 hours of sleep a night, more than half of the weight they lost was fat. But when the volunteers slept just 5.5 hours a night, only one-fourth of the weight lost was fat; the rest of it was mostly muscle tissue.

Also, when the dieters got less sleep, *dieting became impossible.* Their levels of the appetite-promoting hormone ghrelin increased, making the sleep-deprived dieters even hungrier. Getting ample sleep each night may naturally enhance the benefits of any diet plan you are on. Plus, it makes sense that if you are less hungry, it is easier to be compliant so you can see optimal results—a slimmer, trimmer you. Even if you are not actively dieting, getting a good night's sleep will let you greet the day less likely to snack inappropriately and better able to control your hunger, so you will lose weight effortlessly and naturally.

Deprivation Diets and Bad Sleep

It's not news that eating a balanced diet is essential to stay well and prevent disease. Yet the latest research reveals that what we eat also affects our moods—and possibly influences how calm we are when we turn off the bedroom light and finally crawl into bed at night.

The concept of sleep debt has you taking sleep out of your body's bank account during the day and putting it back at night, but in truth, your body is more like a very sophisticated chemistry set. What goes into your body affects the functioning of everything else inside, especially your ability to sleep.

3 KEYS TO LOSING WEIGHT WITH *THE SLEEP DOCTOR'S DIET PLAN*

1. **Eat small meals that are high in protein and fiber every 3 to 4 hours until 7:00 p.m.** The protein-fiber combination will help stabilize your blood sugar, and you won't find yourself starving at dinnertime or bingeing on late-night snacks like you would with fewer meals per day.

2. **Eliminate calorie-laden sodas and juices from your diet.** These calories definitely add up. Substitute mineral water or herbal teas for these drinks. Try flavored water or add a twist of a citrus fruit or a few cucumber slices to plain water. Even zero-calorie soda is not advised, because the carbonation will give you gas and keep you awake or in a light-sleep stage.

3. **Substitute an olive oil cooking spray for butter or margarine.** Using this cooking spray can cut hundreds of calories from each dish you prepare.

Foods to Sleep By

The idea that diet could play a key role in getting good sleep—or not sleeping at all—has been largely ignored by health care professionals. Perhaps the diet-sleep equation was overlooked because most studies on foods' impacts on the body and mind are relatively new. Today, we are learning more about the mechanisms of sleep, what sleep does for the body and mind, and how we can influence sleep with external factors such as foods and natural dietary supplements.

So let's talk turkey—literally. For some time there have been questions about food and sleep. Can food make you sleep? Which foods are sleep-inducing? How does this whole thing work? As always let start with the science:

Foods themselves do not make you sleep. Eating a bowl of tart cherries, which are high in natural melatonin (or drinking the juice; see page 188), will not instantly make you woozy and need to lie down. However, certain foods contain more of particular compounds, and those compounds will interact with your body's natural chemistry to help either start the process of sleep and/or help maintain it.

There are foods in the marketplace that claim to be sleep-inducing. What these are in reality are foods with natural properties that help relax your body, in turn allowing you to fall and stay asleep. The most common sleep-inducing foods are those that contain tryptophan. Tryptophan is an essential amino acid—it cannot be created by the body but must enter the system in the form of food or some other compound.

Amino acids are building blocks for many substances in the body that make the body function.[2] In the case of sleep, tryptophan is a building block for serotonin (a neurotransmitter) that has numerous effects on the human brain. It produces a feeling of relaxation, calmness, and relief from anxiety and depression, all of which may aid sleep. In addition, tryptophan is also one of the building blocks for melatonin. (See pages 58 and 186 to learn more about melatonin.)

Tryptophan—available in most protein and dairy-based foods—can be found in foods such as chocolate, oats, dried dates, milk, yogurt, cottage cheese, red meat, eggs, fish, poultry, sesame seeds, chickpeas, sunflower seeds, pumpkin seeds, spirulina, tofu, and peanuts.

When complex carbohydrates are eaten, they cause the body to release insulin, which not only helps metabolize sugar (glucose) but also removes the amino acids from circulation that compete with tryptophan, allowing it and, eventually, serotonin and melatonin to move into the brain.[3]

Calcium also aids in the process of creating melatonin from tryptophan,[4] as well as magnesium, which plays a role in the creation of serotonin.

In the past 2 decades, hundreds of clinical trials have confirmed a relationship between specific foods and our ability to feel calm and alert. Judith Wurtman, PhD, a nutrition researcher at MIT, has reported that certain foods affect brain chemicals that influence our moods and mental energy and performance.[5] These persuasive foods, such as breads, cereals, pasta, and whole grain crackers, are high in carbohydrates and raise the level of the brain chemical serotonin. As we've discussed, an increased serotonin level in the brain calms you and reduces anxiety, and in some cases promotes drowsiness.

FOODS THAT BOOST SEROTONIN AND CALMNESS

- Almonds
- Bagels
- Black-eyed peas
- Breads
- Cereals
- Cheddar cheese
- Crackers
- Dairy products
- English walnuts
- Gruyère cheese
- Muffins
- Pasta
- Potatoes
- Pumpkin seeds
- Rice
- Sherbet (any flavor)
- Swiss cheese
- Turkey
- Whole grains

Serotonin is the target of a commonly prescribed class of antidepressants called selective serotonin reuptake inhibitors (SSRIs), which increase the amount of serotonin available to the brain and include such drugs as Prozac and Zoloft. Studies have shown that including plenty of foods high in complex carbohydrates in your diet may also boost the level of serotonin, allowing you to reap the benefits of a more relaxed feeling throughout the day as well as sounder sleep.

My patient Sarah had a history of compulsive exercise and deprivation dieting. She eagerly followed every restrictive diet that came along to help her stay trim. Sarah cut back on sleep like she cut calories—but she didn't feel great much of the time. She was really only interested in

SLEEP 101

WAKE UP AND SMELL THE SUGAR PILL . . .

Millions of people use diphenhydramine (Benadryl), a common antihistamine, to lull themselves to sleep (think any of the PM types of pain relievers). Here's a little secret that millions probably don't realize. This common antihistamine works by virtue of its placebo effect. Placebos, sometimes called sugar pills, can include vitamins, herbal supplements, saline infusions, dummy pills, and doses of medicine too low to be effective.

In the world of sleep professionals, Benadryl is considered a placebo when used as a sleep-inducing drug because there is no clinical data to suggest that Benedryl or its active ingredients will help you fall asleep or stay asleep any longer than a sugar pill. And to add insult to injury, the half-life of this medication means you could wake up feeling a bit hungover, as it has similar effects to alcohol.

If Benadryl helps you fall asleep, stick to your story (for the placebo effect), but don't make it a habit or use it all the time. Instead, start to establish better sleep habits as described throughout this book. Talk openly with your physician about your sleep issues and get his or her medical advice.

getting the bare minimum amount of sleep that she absolutely needed, so she could have more time during the rest of the day to exercise, organize, and, in her words, "get the most out of life."

Sarah never realized that what she ate (or didn't) during the day could have a tremendous effect on her sleep (or lack thereof) at night. But as we worked together, she began to learn more about the link between nutrients and sleep. Sarah began to add more serotonin-boosting complex carbs to her diet, especially at bedtime to help induce feelings of calmness and relaxation.

Here are some of my favorite sleep-friendly meals and bedtime snacks.

Meals

- Pasta with Parmesan cheese (avoid tomato-based sauces, since the high acidity can increase the likelihood of reflux)
- Scrambled egg whites and cheese
- Vegetable stir-fry with tofu and brown rice
- Whole wheat pita with hummus (as a side with any lean protein or vegetable dish)
- Seafood, pasta, and cottage cheese
- Meats or poultry with veggies (especially broccoli, spinach, and artichokes)
- Tuna salad sandwich on whole grain bread
- Chili with beans (not spicy) and a sweet potato
- Green salad with tuna chunks and sesame seeds (rich in tryptophan) and whole wheat crackers

Bedtime Snacks

Many of the women I work with are surprised to hear that I often suggest a bedtime snack. After all, doesn't this kind of fly in the face of some of the *Sleep Doctor's 5 Simple Rules?* Yes and no. While I want you to stop eating 3 to 4 hours before bed so that the digestion process is not competing with the sleep induction process, you simply cannot go to bed hungry! Going to bed hungry elevates levels of cortisol, and this stress hormone will keep you awake! If you ate dinner very early or didn't have time for a full evening meal, the benefits of having a small, late night meal outweigh the drawbacks. As always, we are looking to create a balance.

So what does all this mean for your bedtime snack? You will want to find something that has a small amount of protein (which will contain the compounds needed to help produce tryptophan) along with something with enough complex carbohydrates to create insulin (which will take away any competing amino acids and just leave the tryptophan) for a calming, relaxing effect.

My favorite bedtime snacks fall under the category of about 200 or so calories. They should be eaten about 1 to 1½ hours before bed (to allow for digestion) and remember *portion control!*

- A small bowl (1 scoop) of vanilla ice cream or, even better, a frozen soy-based dessert
- A small piece of whole wheat bread with some seed or nut spread (my new favorite is sunbutter, made from sunflower seeds)
- A small bowl of cereal (non-sugar) with low-fat milk and a banana
- Banana and peanut butter on whole wheat toast
- A small amount of grated mozzarella, cheddar, or—better yet—soy cheese, melted under the broiler on a piece of whole wheat bread
- Oatmeal cookies and milk
- A bowl of warm oatmeal with milk and banana
- Yogurt with bananas, almonds, and granola
- Whole wheat English muffin with cream cheese
- Cottage cheese with banana or tart cherries
- Cottage cheese and a small amount of whole wheat pasta
- And my all-time favorite: cheesecake (but make it a small piece)

Food Myths and Facts

In talking with hundreds of patients, I've come to realize that there are a lot of myths about foods out there. Let's look at several common beliefs and I'll explain which ones really work—and which ones do not work when it comes to getting the best sleep.

Statement: "Turkey will put you to sleep because it contains the enzyme tryptophan, which promotes sleep."

Reality: Turkey contains an amino acid called tryptophan, which is a precursor in the synthesis of serotonin in the brain. This means tryptophan is the raw substance the brain uses to manufacture that relaxing neurotransmitter. During the late 1960s and early 1970s, pharmacological studies suggested that the hormone serotonin might have a role in making people feel sleepy. Later on, research in animals showed that destruction of the part of the brain that houses serotonin-producing nerve cells caused total insomnia. And in a study of 50 people with fibromyalgia, an arthritis-like syndrome with symptoms of muscle pain, fatigue, and difficulty sleeping, researchers found that supplementation with 5-hydroxytryptophan (the substance the body makes with tryptophan) improved symptoms of pain, anxiety, and fatigue.[6]

Sure, turkey is "sleep friendly." Yet, while sleep-friendly foods such as turkey may help you relax and fall asleep, *turkey is not a sleeping pill.* For tryptophan to get across the blood–brain barrier and have any effect on your brain, the food containing the amino acid must be ingested by itself on an empty stomach. In fact, chicken and beef contain about the same amount of tryptophan as turkey.

The Bottom Line: You'd likely have to eat about *40 pounds of turkey* to get enough tryptophan to make you sleepy.

Statement: "Taking supplemental tryptophan helps you sleep."

Reality: In addition to occurring naturally in certain foods, tryptophan is available as an over-the-counter dietary supplement that has been used as a sleep aid. However, the evidence is inconclusive about whether taking it in this form is a cure for insomnia.

The Bottom Line: Talk to your doctor before taking any dietary supplement to boost your sleep. Sometimes supplements such as tryptophan can have the opposite effect and cause wakefulness.

Statement: "A high-protein diet may interfere with sleep."

Reality: Eating a high-protein meal without any accompanying carbohydrates can interfere with your sleep. High-protein meals can keep you awake because protein-rich foods contain the amino acid tyrosine, which perks up the brain.

In contrast, if you eat a high-carb meal before bedtime, the resulting rise in blood sugar triggers the pancreas to release a burst of insulin to lower it. In clearing the sugar from your blood, the insulin also clears out the amino acids that compete with tryptophan. More tryptophan can then enter your brain and produce sleep-enhancing compounds such as serotonin and melatonin.

In fact, in a study published in the *American Journal of Clinical Nutrition,* the authors concluded that a meal with a high glycemic index (GI) helps induce sleep because carbohydrates increase the blood's concentration of tryptophan.[7]

The glycemic index is a numerical system that ranks carbohydrates on a scale of 0 to 100 according to their effect on blood glucose (sugar) level. Foods that have no carbohydrates (such as meat, poultry, and fish) have glycemic indexes of zero. A baked potato has a glycemic index of 85. The authors of the *American Journal of Clinical Nutrition* paper found that eating a high-GI meal 4 hours before bed reduced the time it took to fall asleep by 9 minutes. If you experiment with high-GI foods before bedtime to see if they work for you, be sure to watch your calorie intake, or you may add pounds while you add sleep time.

The Bottom Line: Eating small amounts of carbs may help you get to sleep.

Statement: "The best bedtime snack is homemade cookies and milk."

Reality: For a soothing bedtime snack, eat foods that are high in complex carbohydrates along with a tiny amount of protein that contains

DO SPICES AFFECT YOUR SLEEP?

Which spices will lull you to sleep? Which ones will steal your sleep? Whether spices can help or hinder sleep is an interesting question.

Spices have long been known as nature's secret weapons for a variety of human needs. They add much more than just flavor to dishes and drinks. They can impart an enormous number of health benefits as well, from lowering blood sugar and inflammation to boosting digestion and weight loss. Some are touted as antidotes to stress, while others are marketed as anti-aging gems that can make you look and feel younger. (Case in point: Any spice that has antioxidant properties is bound to be sold as a youth restorer.)

When spices are used in a heavy dish—say, a bowl of traditional chili or a rich curry—the effects of all that food on the stomach and digestion can put a kink in your sound sleep regardless of the spices involved.

Most of us need at least 4 hours to digest a meal like that. If you hit the hay too soon, you're confusing your body—creating a tug-of-war between its need to activate itself to digest and your attempt to fall asleep. And anyone who struggles with heartburn, or GERD, knows that consuming a large, spicy meal before bedtime is asking for trouble.

But not all spices are, in fact, *spicy.* Consider the following:

- **Nutmeg, turmeric, and garlic** have been shown to *promote* sleep.
- **Herbs** such as parsley, dill, sage, and basil are thought to promote sleep and reduce insomnia.

Scientists around the world continue to search for clues to explain how spices affect our health and, in particular, our sleep. If you're looking to "spice up your sleep life" to get a good night's sleep, I suggest the following:

- **Cook with sleep-friendly herbs** such as parsley, dill, sage, and basil whenever possible.
- **Watch out for heavy, fatty dishes** that can make late-night digestion tough. No amount of sleep-friendly spices can counter the effects of too much fat and protein that make for difficult digestion.
- **Drink herbal tea blended with spices** before bedtime, such as those with cloves or nutmeg. (Avoid caffeine.)

just enough tryptophan to soothe and relax your brain. Include some calcium, too, because this mineral helps the brain use the tryptophan to make the serotonin from which melatonin is manufactured. This explains why dairy products, which contain both tryptophan and calcium, are one of the top sleep-inducing foods.

The Bottom Line: While homemade cookies may be tempting, the perfect bedtime snack may be a slice of whole grain toast with a light spread of peanut butter and a small glass of low-fat milk.

Statement: "A glass of warm milk is the best sleep medicine you can take."

Reality: Warm milk seems to help some individuals fall asleep. Perhaps people relate warm milk to childhood memories of Mom serving them cookies and milk before bedtime! But there is not a lot of evidence to show that there is anything in the milk in sufficient quantity to help with sleep.

The Bottom Line: While tryptophan is present in milk, you would need to drink about a gallon to get enough to make any difference, and then you would be waking up repeatedly all night to urinate. So, no, warm milk in itself does not have a somnolent effect—but the comforting memories of childhood days might.

Statement: "You won't sleep well if you go to bed hungry."

Reality: If you experience hunger pangs at night, you should have a snack close to bedtime (about an hour before). That snack should be from the complex carbohydrate category, such as a piece of whole grain toast with a thin spread of natural peanut butter or a slice of reduced-fat cheese on top.

Another good choice is a banana. Bananas combine sleep-inducing melatonin, calming serotonin, and muscle-relaxing magnesium.

The Bottom Line: Bedtime snacks should be consumed about an hour before your actual bedtime and be under 200 calories—no more. If you eat a food containing tryptophan before bedtime, allow about an hour for the amino acid to reach your brain. In other words, don't wait until right before you hop in bed to have your snack.

5 WAYS TO SLEEP WELL AND LOSE WEIGHT

1. **Substitute whole grains for white flour products.** The additional fiber will improve your health and keep you feeling full for a longer period of time.

2. **Do not eat after 7:00 p.m. unless you eat a light bedtime snack.** If you must have a bedtime snack, choose something light like low-fat yogurt with a sprinkling of chopped walnuts or granola, a small bowl of oatmeal made with fat-free milk, or a piece of whole grain toast with 1 teaspoon of peanut butter. (See my bedtime-snack list on page 174.)

3. **Choose nighttime snacks that contain complex carbohydrates, a limited amount of protein, and calcium.** Dairy products are great sleep inducers because the brain can use their calcium and trypto-phan to manufacture melatonin. Adding carbohydrates to dairy or protein calms us down with a serotonin buzz. However, make sure you don't consume too much protein close to bedtime. Otherwise, you might get too much energy from the amino acid tyrosine, which perks you up. *Try to keep your bedtime snack under 200 calories,* and avoid foods that might induce heartburn, like spicy or garlicky foods.

4. **Avoid eating high-protein meals too close to bedtime.** Eating a meal high in carbohydrates stimulates the release of insulin, which helps clear the bloodstream of amino acids that compete with the amino acid tryptophan. This allows more of that natural sleep-inducing amino acid to enter the brain and be used to manufacture sleep-inducing substances such as serotonin and melatonin. Remember, eating a high-protein meal without any accompanying carbohydrates may keep you wide awake from the tyrosine, which perks up the brain.

5. **Avoid eating sleep busters too close to bedtime,** including spicy foods, tomato sauce, carbonated drinks, citrus, chocolate, fatty and fried foods, garlic and onions, mint, and anything with caffeine as an ingredient.

Nutritional Building Blocks for Great Sleep

Your body's need for vitamins and minerals increases under certain conditions, such as chronic stress. When these essential nutrients are unavailable for daily functioning, your body gets worn down. When this happens, you are at risk for health problems, including poor sleep. Be sure to talk with your doctor before you take any vitamins or minerals just to make sure they don't interact with medications you are taking. Also, some people are highly stimulated by B vitamins, so try taking these vitamins early in the day to see how you react. *Some foods that are high in B vitamins include whole grains, cereals, nuts, potatoes, and broccoli.*

Here are the vitamins and minerals that I believe are essential to getting good sleep each night.

Vitamin B. The B vitamins are vital in regulating your body's use of tryptophan and other amino acids. Because stress, smoking, alcohol, and environmental factors can rob you of B vitamins, sometimes you need to rely on supplements in order to get an adequate supply.

Vitamin B_3 (niacin) has been found to increase the effectiveness of tryptophan. Some studies suggest that B_3 lengthens REM sleep and decreases the time an insomniac is awake at night. What's more, vitamin B_3 has been used to treat mood disorders such as depression. If depression is effectively treated, it is much easier to get to sleep and stay asleep. Vitamin B_3 also helps with blood sugar balance, which can help with sleep (and control hunger).[8]

Vitamin B_6 is required for the production of serotonin, the calming neurotransmitter that helps to modulate your mood, hunger, sleep patterns, and sensitivity to pain.[9]

CHAMOMILE TEA FOR SLEEP

For thousands of years, people have used chamomile medicinally. The tea and essential oil have been used for their calming effects and for insomnia relief.

One Japanese study of sleep-disturbed rats found that chamomile extract helped the rats drift off to sleep more quickly—and just as quickly as the rats that received a dose of a benzodiazepine (a tranquilizer).

A few precautions: If you have an allergy to ragweed, don't use chamomile. Also avoid it if you are pregnant, because it may act as a uterine stimulant, or when breastfeeding, because its effect on nursing babies hasn't been well studied. And obviously, you shouldn't use chamomile when driving, because it may cause drowsiness.

In addition, chamomile may increase the risk of bleeding, so people taking blood thinners should exercise caution. Chamomile may also increase blood pressure.

Vitamin B$_{12}$ appears to help some women regain normal sleep patterns after bouts of insomnia and frequent awakenings during the night. By acting on the pineal gland, B$_{12}$ triggers a faster release of melatonin.[10]

Folic acid deficiency can cause insomnia, so having a sufficient supply is key. In addition, all women of childbearing age who may become pregnant need at least 400 micrograms of folic acid daily to prevent neural tube defects in the fetus.

Vitamin D is a fat-soluble vitamin, but it actually functions as a hormone in the body. The most readily available source of vitamin D is your body's production of it in response to sunlight, which is the reason that getting 15 minutes of sunlight per day is one of the *Sleep Doctor's 5 Simple Rules* for weight loss through better sleep. If you don't get

SLEEPY-TIME HERBS AND NATURAL DIETARY SUPPLEMENTS

Some natural supplements and herbs such as valerian, S-adenosylmethionine (SAMe), and 5-hydroxytryptophan (5-HTP), which the body makes from tryptophan)[11] claim to promote sleep. These supplements are available over the counter, but buyer beware! The FDA does not regulate natural supplements, so the safety, contents, quality, and effectiveness of these supplements are not well studied or monitored. Natural supplements can interact with other drugs, as well as with alcohol. Also, pregnant or breastfeeding women should not take them.[12, 13]

The National Institutes of Health and the National Center for Complementary and Alternative Medicine (NCCAM) put out a "quick guide" to herbs that I find highly useful in my clinic.[14] You can download it in PDF format from the Web site, http://nccam.nih.gov, where you can also find valuable information on complementary and alternative medicine.

In the chart here, I have listed the herbs and natural supplements historically used for sleep and these organizations' assessments of the reliability of the research and possible side effects.

HERB	SCIENCE	SIDE EFFECTS
CHAMOMILE (GERMAN)	Not a lot of scientific substantiation of claims; more anecdotal reports. Still, many claim effectiveness.	If you are allergic to ragweed, use caution. Otherwise, chamomile is generally safe.
KAVA	Some scientific evidence for use as an anxiety reducer	Liver damage, including liver failure
LAVENDER	Some evidence for use as an anxiety reducer; more effective as an aromatherapy agent	Lavender oil applied to the skin can cause irritation; if ingested, the oil can be poisonous.
L-TRYPTOPHAN AND 5-HTP	Have not been proven effective	May be linked to eosinophilia-myalgia syndrome, a systemic condition that causes severe muscle pain and changes in the blood
VALERIAN	Some data support the use of valerian for insomnia.	May cause dizziness, but generally safe for short-term use

enough vitamin D, supplements may be necessary. Vitamin D helps to activate calcium and phosphorus in the bloodstream. When the body has an insufficient supply of vitamin D, the blood levels of calcium and phosphorus plummet, as well. Your body then turns to the bones to replenish the calcium. Deficiencies of the minerals calcium and phosphorus are directly linked to osteoporosis and a host of other bone-weakening problems. There are numerous findings showing that vitamin D is an important nutrient for multiple facets of health, including insulin function, cancer prevention (especially of the breast, colon, and prostate), and cardiovascular health. Although younger adults tend to get sufficient sunlight throughout the day to keep this vitamin in good supply, many middle-aged and older adults do not. Studies show that aging reduces the skin's ability to make use of sunlight to manufacture vitamin D.[15] Consequently, daily vitamin D supplements of 800 IU from ages 65 to 70 are suggested. Some experts suggest that men and women over 50 should take 800 IU of vitamin D year-round.

The usual recommended dietary allowance for vitamin D is 400 IU. Along with sunlight, you can also obtain this bone-strengthening vitamin from food sources such as halibut-liver oil, herring, cod-liver oil, mackerel, salmon, tuna, fortified milk, and fortified cereals. So talk with your doctor to see if you should consider supplementing your vitamin D intake.

Calcium is a natural relaxer that has a calming effect on the nervous system. Most women do not get enough calcium in their diets, especially if they are watching their calories. Take calcium in 500-milligram (mg) or smaller doses between meals. *Foods high in calcium include dairy products, salmon with bones, sardines, calcium-enriched juices and other food products, soy foods, and leafy green vegetables.*

Magnesium may boost good-quality sleep, whether you are a chronic insomniac or experience poor sleep only on occasion. If you try magnesium as a sleep aid, be sure to take it in balanced proportions of two parts calcium to one part magnesium (but do not take more than 350 mg magnesium a day). *Foods high in magnesium include cereals, nuts, sunflower seeds, tofu, dairy products, bananas, pineapple, raisins, artichokes, avocados, lima beans, oysters, halibut, grouper, cod, and sole.*

Zinc deficiency is linked to insomnia, so be sure to get ample zinc in the foods you eat each day. *Good choices include baked beans, chicken, eggs, fortified cereals, lean pork, lean red meat, low-fat milk and yogurt, oysters and other shellfish, tofu, and turkey.*

Copper and iron deficiencies can seriously affect your sleep. Iron deficiency is known to be a trigger of restless legs syndrome. In fact, I have had several patients whose weird feelings in their legs simply vanished after they started a regimen of iron supplementation. *Foods high in iron include dried apricots, dried beans, enriched or fortified breads and cereals, lentils, lean red meat, prunes, and raisins. Foods high in copper include beef, oysters, beans, sunflower seeds, tofu, soy milk, potatoes, and sweet potatoes.*

How should you get all these sleepy-time vitamins and minerals? I believe that most women can take in adequate amounts of these nutrients by eating whole foods. In addition, a good multivitamin should contain all these vitamins and minerals. If you feel you need to supplement with more than just the recommended dietary allowances, talk

MOVING AROUND TOO MUCH AT NIGHT?

If you are iron deficient, you may have restless legs syndrome (see page 35), which can cause you to wake up frequently and feel exhausted the next day. A simple blood test is used to determine how much stored iron your body has. Any level below 60 nanograms per milliliter could indicate an iron issue but still be in the normal range and the source of your restlessness. But be careful: Supplemental iron taken in large doses can cause constipation. Ask your doctor about an iron supplement and be sure to include plenty of iron-rich foods such as red meat, spinach, and broccoli in your diet.

with your doctor. You want to make sure you supplement safely and don't get too much of any essential vitamin or mineral.

Soy Foods May Reduce Night Sweats

If you have hormone-related night sweats or hot flashes that interrupt your sleep, you may want to eat more foods that contain phytoestrogens. These plant-derived compounds mimic estrogen in the body. The most common phytoestrogens are isoflavones, flavones, and lignins.

The phytoestrogens in soy perform some of the same actions in the body that the hormone estrogen does, and they appear to have few harmful side effects. Some women believe that soy helps relieve the menopausal symptoms that frequently result from plummeting estrogen levels. (If you have estrogen-dependent breast cancer, talk to your doctor before eating any soy products.)

For years, soybeans have played an integral part in the Asian diet. In fact, heart disease, breast cancer, prostate cancer, and osteoporosis rates for Asian men and women are much lower than they are for Americans. An easy way to include phytoestrogens in your diet is to eat more soy foods. Soy, the most complete vegetable protein, is rich in vitamin E, fiber, calcium, magnesium, lecithin, riboflavin, thiamin, folic acid, and iron.

Some top soy favorites include:

- Roasted soy nuts
- Edamame
- Tempeh
- Tofu
- Soy cheese
- Soy ice cream
- Soy milk

IS MELATONIN A NATURAL SLEEP MIRACLE?

I get a lot of questions about melatonin, especially since many supplement companies and health food stores promote melatonin as a "natural" sleep aid. Given the availability of this natural dietary supplement today, you'd assume that melatonin is both safe and effective. But let's look further.

Melatonin is a sleep regulator, not a sleep initiator. Melatonin is a **hormone** your body produces to help regulate your sleep-wake cycle, among other functions, but melatonin does not make you fall asleep. Melatonin is **not** a vitamin or mineral. When the sun sets and darkness falls, a pea-size structure located deep between the hemispheres of your brain called the pineal gland begins to secrete melatonin—preparing you for sleep. (Melatonin is also secreted in the GI tract for other nonsleep reasons.)

As the melatonin level in the blood rises, you start to feel less alert and sleepier. The melatonin level stays elevated for about 12 hours, falling back to the low daytime level by about 9:00 a.m. The daytime level of melatonin is barely detectable.

The precise mechanism of melatonin secretion is not well understood. We do know, however, that melatonin isn't just about the sleep-wake cycle. It has also been shown to have the following functions.

- Helps to regulate the female reproductive cycle
- Controls the onset of puberty; children who take melatonin can have delayed sexual development, so never, ever give a child a melatonin supplement
- Helps to regulate bloodflow, specifically by constricting the coronary arteries
- Increases depression in people prone to this illness

Now, taking any hormone with all these possible effects—even one that is "natural"—is something you should consider only after discussing it with your doctor. Warning: Melatonin should **never** be given to children, meaning anyone under the age of 18 should not take it.

Most commercial melatonin products are offered at overdosage levels that cause the melatonin in the blood to rise to a much higher level than is naturally produced in the body. Taking a typical dose of melatonin (1 to 3 mg) may elevate your blood melatonin level to 1 to 20 times the normal state. ***The correct dosage is between 0.3 and 0.5 milligrams (mg).*** In addition, if you take melatonin at the wrong time of day, you may reset your biological clock in an undesirable direction.

How much to take, when to take it, and how effective it is, if at all, for particular sleep disorders is only beginning to be understood. OTC melatonin comes to the brain in a large burst, not like the normal slow rise and fall so its effects will be different. Speak to your doctor about possible interactions that melatonin could have with your other medications. Remember, melatonin is like a signal to your brain that nightfall has come. The general recommendations for the use of melatonin include:

- If you are having sleep problems meaning that you sleep well just at the wrong time, consider taking melatonin about 90 minutes before your desired bedtime, supervised by a sleep specialist.
- Melatonin should not be taken for more than 2 weeks.
- You should not expose yourself to bright light after taking melatonin, or your brain will get two conflicting signals that may result in insomnia!

I recommend regulating your own sleep-wake cycle in a genuinely natural way by:

- Exposing yourself to light during the day (preferably sunlight)
- Engaging in physical activity regularly
- Practicing good sleep hygiene

Your body will reset its internal clock with the proper exposure to light at the right time. You shouldn't take an over-the-counter nighttime pain reliever either, unless you truly do need to ease muscle aches or other pain that might prevent you from going to sleep easily. But don't make taking melatonin your nightly habit instead.

Besides tofu, over the past decade more than 2,000 new soy products have been introduced to consumers, including meatless pepperoni, salami, hot dogs, and bacon as well as puddings and dairy alternatives. You can also find calcium-rich soy foods such as calcium-set tofu, fortified soy milk, textured vegetable protein, and soy nuts.

The Future Is Bright for Better Sleep

With groundbreaking studies surfacing daily on sleep and its link with overweight and obesity, the future is very bright for finding new ways to resolve sleeplessness, get better sleep, and manage your weight. Whatever you do to improve your sleep and lose weight, I urge you to follow

NEW SLEEP RESEARCH ALERT: TART CHERRY JUICE AND MELATONIN

There are lots of drinks that are marketed as doing something healthy for you. Drink orange juice if you have a cold. Try cranberry juice to keep your urinary tract healthy. Pomegranate juice is touted for its age-defying antioxidants. Sip milk to get more calcium to build strong bones. But what about a daily drink to help you sleep? Something made from fruit? And something other than the storied nightcap of sleep-disrupting alcohol? A new study by a team from the University of Rochester in New York found that **tart cherry juice** might be the answer.[16]

The researchers looked at the sleep of 15 older adults who drank 8 ounces of tart cherry juice in the morning and evening for 2 weeks. Then they drank a placebo with no tart cherry juice for another 2-week period. The result? A significant **reduction in reported severity of insomnia during the weeks when they drank the cherry juice.** The adults experienced about 17 fewer minutes awake after initially going to sleep, on average, when they drank the cherry juice.

So what's the magic in cherry juice? **Cherries contain melatonin!** So, getting **natural melatonin from whole foods** like cherries is clearly a good option in sleep medicine.

your doctor's advice. In this book, I've demonstrated how sleep loss leads to weight gain and how you can take control of your sleep and, in turn, take better control of your weight. You now have the *Sleep Doctor's 5 Simple Rules* that you can use with *any* diet plan or nutritional program to help with sleep and weight loss. And you now better understand how to find products that can help you sleep by meeting your sleep needs. In addition, we have discussed hands-on tools to decrease your stress before bed and some strategies for coping with situations that can disrupt your sleep (kids, travel, snoring, you name it!).

I know this book will help you to sleep and lose the weight you want to, to help you lead a happier and healthier life. Remember: Everything you do . . . you will do better with a good night's sleep.

Part III

The Sleep Doctor's DIET PLAN RECIPES

T*he Sleep Doctor's Diet Plan* recipes are made with the same calming foods and nutrients discussed in Chapter 8. For instance, complex carbohydrates found in fruits, vegetables, and whole grains can trigger the production of serotonin in the brain. Serotonin, a neurotransmitter, produces a calming effect and may help you feel relaxed for a period of time. Foods such as salmon and dairy products are high in calcium, which is a natural relaxant that has a calming effect on the nervous system. Your brain uses calcium and the amino acid tryptophan to manufacture melatonin, the sleep hormone. This is why dairy products are great sleep boosters. When you add some carbs to dairy such as with a **Banana Smoothie (page 200),** you increase calming serotonin in your body. Other foods high in magnesium are natural relaxers and important for good sleep.

Whether you are a meat eater, a vegetarian, or someone who wants to "eat to sleep," these recipes will help you to relax, get good sleep, and finally lose weight.

Snacks

Parmesan Cheese Toasts

Who says you can't enjoy cheese toast before bed? This yummy snack is comforting, filling, and flavorful with the dash of Italian herb seasoning.

1	**whole wheat baguette (about 15 inches)**
¼	**cup olive oil**
½	**teaspoon Italian herb seasoning**
1	**cup grated Parmesan cheese**

Preheat the oven to 350°F. Cut the baguette on a slight diagonal into slices about ½ inch thick.

In a small bowl, combine the oil and Italian seasoning. Brush both sides of the bread slices with the oil mixture. Place on a baking sheet and bake for 7 minutes. Turn the slices over and sprinkle the Parmesan on top. Bake until the edges are crisp and the cheese has melted and is lightly browned, about 5 minutes.

Serves 6

Per serving: 173 calories, 14 g fat (4 g saturated), 12 mg cholesterol, 288 mg sodium, 8 g total carbohydrates (1 g sugars), 1.5 g fiber, 8 g protein

Roasted Pepper Hummus

Eating the proper ratio of protein and carbs is important to feeling relaxed. Spread the roasted pepper hummus on half of a whole-grain bagel for a delicious, full-flavor "lite" meal or bedtime snack.

1¾	cups cooked chickpeas
½	cup roasted red peppers
⅓	cup tahini
3	large cloves garlic, smashed and peeled
3	tablespoons fresh lemon juice
3	tablespoons extra-virgin olive oil
1	teaspoon ground cumin
1	teaspoon salt
⅛	teaspoon ground black pepper
	Pinch of ground red pepper

Combine the chickpeas, red peppers, tahini, garlic, lemon juice, oil, cumin, salt, black pepper, and ground red pepper in a food processor. Process until smooth and creamy. Season with additional salt and black pepper, if desired.

Serves 16

Per serving: 71 calories, 3.5 g fat (0.5 g saturated), 0 mg cholesterol, 152 mg sodium, 8 g total carbohydrates (2 g sugars), 2.5 g fiber, 3 g protein

Roasted Lemon-Herb Tofu

Need a quick dinner but want to avoid take-out? The roasted lemon-herb tofu is a healthy, low-calorie source of protein that's easy to make and yummy, too. Add a mixed green salad and a slice of whole-grain bread for a complete meal.

2	packages (15 ounces each) extra-firm tofu
2	tablespoons fresh lemon juice
1	tablespoon extra-virgin olive oil
1	clove garlic, finely minced
2	tablespoons loosely packed fresh basil leaves, chopped
2	teaspoons fresh oregano leaves, chopped
1	teaspoon fresh rosemary leaves, chopped
1	teaspoon coarse salt

Drain the tofu for 30 minutes (see tip below).

Preheat the oven to 375°F.

Stir together the lemon juice, oil, garlic, basil, oregano, rosemary, and salt in a small bowl. Pat the tofu pieces dry and brush them all over with the herb mixture. Roast for 45 to 50 minutes, flipping occasionally, until browned and hot.

Serves 4

Per serving: 228 calories, 16 g fat (1.5 g saturated), 0 mg cholesterol, 498 mg sodium, 6 g total carbohydrates (1.5 g sugars), 1 g fiber, 21 g protein

TIP Draining excess liquid from tofu makes it much sturdier for adding to stir-fries and soups. It also makes the tofu more receptive to absorbing flavorful marinades. Cut a block of tofu in half horizontally. Then cut each piece in half crosswise to make rectangles roughly 3¼ x 2¼ inches. Arrange the tofu pieces in an even layer on a baking sheet. Prop the baking sheet up at one end by at least an inch (more if possible) and have the other end overhang the sink. Cover with 2 thicknesses of paper towel and top with another baking sheet or a cutting board. Weight down with a heavy skillet or a few cans. Let the tofu drain into the sink for at least 30 minutes.

Apples with Honey-Yogurt Dip and Candied Walnuts

This comforting snack may remind you of childhood when mom served milk and warm cookies before bed. The carb-protein ratio of the apples, walnuts, and Greek yogurt will help you sleep like a baby.

1	teaspoon sugar
1	tablespoon hot water
2	tablespoons walnuts
⅓	cup fat-free plain Greek yogurt
1	tablespoon honey
1	apple, sliced

Combine the sugar and water in a small bowl and stir to dissolve the sugar.

Place the walnuts in a small skillet and cook over medium-high heat, shaking the pan often, until lightly toasted, 3 to 5 minutes. Remove the skillet from the heat and stir in the sugar mixture, tossing to coat. Let cool.

Place the yogurt in a small bowl and cover with the honey and walnuts. Serve with apple slices for dipping.

Serves 1

Per serving: 266 calories, 8 g fat (1 g saturated), 2 mg cholesterol, 47 mg sodium, 49 g total carbohydrates (41 g sugars), 3 g fiber, 6 g protein

Cheese and Crackers

Cottage cheese provides you with carbohydrates, protein, and calcium—the important nutritional trio for feeling calm at bedtime. A simple snack of cottage cheese, olives, and crackers help fill you up before bed so cravings won't disrupt your sleep.

½	cup low fat cottage cheese
1	cup chopped red bell pepper
10	large black olives
1	teaspoon salt-free Italian seasoning
6	Ry-Krisp crackers

Mix the cottage cheese, bell pepper, olives, and Italian seasoning. Serve with the crackers.

Serves 1

Per serving: 355 calories, 6 g fat (1 g saturated), 5 mg cholesterol, 555 mg sodium, 58 g total carbohydrates (5 g sugars), 2 g fiber, 18 g protein

Apple-Cinnamon Yogurt

Rare is the woman who can climb into bed and fall asleep instantly. This comforting apple-cinnamon yogurt is an easy treat that boasts carbohydrates, which have a calming, drowsiness-inducing effect, and lots of flavor.

1	small apple, chopped
2	tablespoons chopped walnuts
1	teaspoon honey (optional)
⅛	teaspoon ground cinnamon
½	cup fat-free plain yogurt

Place the apple and walnuts in a microwaveable bowl. Top with the honey, if using, and cinnamon. Microwave on high power for 1 minute, or until warmed. Top with the yogurt.

Serves 1

Per serving: 301 calories, 10 g fat (1 g saturated), 2 mg cholesterol, 86 mg sodium, 48 g total carbohydrates (41 g sugars), 4.5 g fiber, 9 g protein

Blueberry-Peanut Butter Shake

When you complement these high-antioxidant berries with some protein and calcium, you get a natural elixir that tastes great and boosts drowsiness

2	**cups fat-free milk**
2	**tablespoons ground flaxseeds**
2	**tablespoons natural no-salt-added creamy peanut butter**
1	**cup frozen blueberries**

Combine the milk, flaxseeds, peanut butter, and blueberries in a blender. Blend until smooth.

Serves 2

Per serving: 253 calories, 10 g fat (1 g saturated), 5 mg cholesterol, 164 mg sodium, 29 g total carbohydrates (20 g sugars), 6 g fiber, 14 g protein

Banana Smoothie

Dairy foods are natural relaxants, which makes yogurt-based smoothies a good choice. Easy to make and an all-time favorite, this sleep-boosting banana smoothie is filled with the perfect carb-protein ratio you need to feel drowsy before bed.

1	container (6 ounces) low-fat vanilla yogurt
½	ripe banana, coarsely chopped
½	cup fat-free milk
¼	teaspoon pure vanilla extract
¼	graham cracker, crushed

Combine the yogurt, banana, milk, and vanilla extract in a blender. Blend until smooth. Pour into a glass. Sprinkle with the graham cracker.

Serves 1

Per serving: 249 calories, 2.5 g fat (1.5 g saturated), 11 mg cholesterol, 175 mg sodium, 45 g total carbohydrates (37 g sugars), 1.5 g fiber, 13 g protein

Mango-Soy Smoothie

Keep your blender on the counter to whip up this mango-soy smoothie before bedtime. The blend of the tart soy yogurt with the tropical mango and orange juice is guaranteed to fill your tummy and give you sweet dreams.

1	container (6 ounces) plain soy yogurt
1	mango, cut into large chunks (about 1 cup)
½	cup orange juice
½	teaspoon ground ginger
½	teaspoon ground cardamom
5	ice cubes

Combine the yogurt, mango, orange juice, ginger, cardamom, and ice in a blender. Puree until thick and smooth.

Serves 2

Per serving: 143 calories, 1.5 g fat (0 g saturated), 0 mg cholesterol, 16 mg sodium, 33 g total carbohydrates (25 g sugars), 3 g fiber, 3 g protein

Entrées

Pork Loin Stuffed with Apricots and Wild Rice

Eating meals with the correct ratio of carbs to protein, like this colorful dish, can boost relaxation and help you feel drowsy at night. Pair this with some steamed or lightly sautéed greens.

Pork Loin

³/₄	cup wild rice
1½	teaspoons olive oil
1	onion, chopped
1	celery rib, chopped
1	garlic clove, minced
1	teaspoon dried thyme
¼	cup Madeira or fat-free chicken broth
½	cup chopped dried apricots
	Salt and ground black pepper
1	pork tenderloin (1½ pounds)

Sauce

1	cup fat-free chicken broth
⅓	cup apricot nectar or orange juice
2	teaspoons Dijon mustard
2	teaspoons cornstarch
2	tablespoons water

To make the pork loin: Prepare the wild rice according to package directions. Meanwhile, heat the oil in a large nonstick skillet over medium heat. Add the onion, celery, garlic, and thyme and cook, stirring frequently, until the onion is soft, 6 to 8 minutes. Add the Madeira or broth and increase the heat to high. Cook until the liquid is evaporated, about 2 minutes. Remove from the heat and stir in the apricots and wild rice. Season with salt and pepper.

Preheat the oven to 350°F. With a knife, make a 1-inch slit from one end of the pork to the other, keeping the sides intact. Push the meat back from the slit to create a "tunnel." From both ends, stuff the cavity with the rice mixture. Mist the pork with cooking spray and season with salt and pepper.

Coat a large ovenproof skillet with cooking spray and heat over medium-high heat. Add the pork and cook until browned on all sides, about 4 minutes. Place the skillet in the oven and bake for 25 minutes, or until a thermometer inserted in the center reaches 155°F and the juices run clear. Let stand for 5 minutes before slicing.

To make the sauce: Whisk together the broth, apricot nectar, or orange juice, and mustard in a small saucepan. Bring to a boil over medium-high heat and cook for 2 minutes. Stir 2 tablespoons water into the cornstarch in a small bowl or cup. Add to the saucepan and cook, whisking, until thickened, about 2 minutes. Serve over the pork.

Serves 1

Per serving: 430 calories, 8 g fat (2 g saturated), 111 mg cholesterol, 319 mg sodium, 44 g total carbohydrates (15 g sugars), 4 g fiber, 42 g protein

Turkey Piccata

Sure, turkey has tryptophan. But you'd have to eat many servings of this piccata to get enough of this sleep-inducing amino acid. Fortunately, there are plenty of other reasons to try it: The turkey piccata is tangy and plenty low in calories and can help you maintain a normal weight—important for getting good sleep. Invest in a high-quality nonstick skillet so that you can cook turkey and chicken cutlets without having to add a lot of extra fat.

2	lemons
⅓	cup all-purpose flour
½	teaspoon ground black pepper
¼	teaspoon salt
1	pound turkey breast, cut into ¼-inch-thick slices
2	teaspoons olive oil
2	cups sliced mushrooms
1	shallot, minced
1	large garlic clove, minced
¼	cup dry vermouth or nonalcoholic white wine
¾	cup fat-free, reduced-sodium chicken broth
2	tablespoons capers, rinsed and drained
¼	teaspoon sugar
2	tablespoons chopped flat-leaf parsley
1	teaspoon unsalted butter or margarine

With a sharp knife, carefully remove the peel and white membrane from one of the lemons. Cut the lemon segments away from their surrounding membranes and place in a small bowl. Squeeze any juice from the membranes into the bowl. Discard the peel, membranes, and seeds. Thinly slice the remaining whole lemon.

Combine the flour, pepper, and salt on a large plate. Dredge the turkey in the flour mixture to coat both sides and shake off any excess. Heat the oil in a large nonstick skillet over medium-high heat. Working in batches if necessary, add the turkey to the skillet and cook until no longer pink in the center, about 2 minutes per side. Transfer to a platter.

Coat the skillet with cooking spray and add the mushrooms, shallot, and garlic. Reduce the heat to medium, cover, and cook for 2 minutes, stirring occasionally. Add the vermouth or wine and increase the heat to medium-high. Bring to a boil and stir constantly for 30 seconds. Add the broth, capers, sugar, and the lemon segments (with juice). Return to a boil and cook for 1 to 2 minutes. Return the turkey to the skillet and add the parsley, butter or margarine, and the lemon slices. Cook and stir until heated through, about 1 minute.

Serves 4

Per serving: 232 calories, 4 g fat (1 g saturated), 48 mg cholesterol, 463 mg sodium, 15 g total carbohydrates (2 g sugars), 2 g fiber, 31 g protein

Turkey Stuffed with Mushrooms and Spinach

The mild flavor of turkey makes it companionable with many flavorings. In this preparation, earthy mushrooms and spinach add depth of flavor.

1	turkey London broil (about 1½ pounds)
2	teaspoons olive oil plus extra for misting
1	cup brown or white mushrooms, chopped
1	cup (1 ounce) baby spinach leaves
½	cup sliced scallions
¼	teaspoon poultry seasoning
⅛	teaspoon salt
	Ground black pepper
2	tablespoons (½ ounce) shredded Swiss cheese

Preheat the oven to 350°F.

Heat 2 teaspoons of the oil in an ovenproof skillet over medium heat. Add the mushrooms, spinach, scallions, poultry seasoning, salt, and pepper to taste. Cook, stirring, until the spinach wilts, about 3 minutes. Set aside to cool for 10 minutes.

Butterfly the turkey by using a sharp knife to cut horizontally through the breast. Open it flat like a book. Spoon the mushroom mixture onto one side of the turkey and top. with the cheese. Fold the other side of the turkey breast over the filling and press the edge to seal. Fasten with toothpicks, if desired.

Add ½ cup of water to the skillet. Bring to a boil over medium heat, scraping with a spatula to release the browned bits on the pan bottom. Off the heat, place the turkey in the skillet. Mist the top of the turkey lightly with olive oil. Roast for 45 minutes, or until a thermometer inserted in the center registers 165°F. Transfer to a cutting board and let stand for 15 minutes, until the internal temperature rises to 170°F. Slice the turkey. Reheat the juices in the skillet to drizzle over the turkey.

Serves 6

Per serving: 150 calories, 4 g fat (0.5 g saturated), 47 mg cholesterol, 127 mg sodium, 1.5 g total carbohydrates (0.5 g sugars), 0.5 g fiber, 29 g protein

Chicken Pasta Niçoise

This hearty chicken pasta Niçoise gets the vote for favorite flavors. The lean chicken, fresh vegetables, and filling pasta smothered in a home-made Italian sauce will leave you super satisfied all night long.

1¼	cups white wine or fat-free chicken broth
2	skinless, bone-in chicken breast halves
2	skinless, bone-in chicken thighs
1	tablespoon minced garlic
½	cup sliced onion
1	can (15 ounces) whole peeled tomatoes, chopped (with juice)
1	cup sliced red bell pepper
1	cup sliced green bell pepper
5	Niçoise olives, pitted and chopped
1	tablespoon Italian herb seasoning
½	pound fettucine or other wide pasta

In a 10-inch nonstick skillet, bring the wine or broth to a boil over medium-high heat. Add the chicken and cook until opaque on both sides.

Add the garlic, onion, tomatoes (with juice), bell peppers, olives, and Italian seasoning. Reduce the heat to medium and cook until the chicken is no longer pink in the center, about 30 minutes.

While the chicken cooks, bring a large pot of salted water to a boil. Add the pasta and cook according to package directions. Drain well.

Divide the pasta among 4 plates and serve topped with the chicken, vegetables, and sauce.

Serves 8

Per serving: 192 calories, 5.5 g fat (1.5 g saturated), 39 mg cholesterol, 240 mg sodium, 38 g total carbohydrates (3.5 g sugars), 3 g fiber, 5 g protein

Chicken Breasts
with Pine Nuts and Tangerines

Looking for guilt-free comfort food? Then try this recipe. The combination of citrus, scallions, and garlic adds a tropical taste to this low-calorie dish.

4	skinless, boneless chicken breast halves (5 ounces each)
2	tablespoons butter
1	tablespoon vegetable oil
1	large garlic clove, minced
½	cup pine nuts
6	tablespoons orange juice
2	scallions (green tops only), chopped
1	tangerine, separated into segments

Place the chicken breasts between 2 pieces of wax paper and pound with the flat side of a meat pounder or a small heavy skillet to even them out.

Heat the butter and oil in a large skillet over medium-high heat. Add the chicken and cook until they just begin to brown slightly, about 2 minutes per side. Transfer to a plate. Add the garlic and pine nuts to the skillet and cook until the pine nuts just begin to brown. Remove from the heat, but while it is still hot, add 3 tablespoons of the orange juice. Stir it around the bottom of the skillet, scraping up all the browned bits. Add the scallion greens.

Return the chicken to the skillet and spoon the pine nut mixture on top. Add the remaining 3 tablespoons orange juice. Cover the skillet and return to low heat for about 5 minutes. Add the tangerine segments and cook until the chicken is cooked through, about 3 minutes. Serve the chicken topped with the tangerines and pine nut sauce.

Serves 4

Per serving: 375 calories, 23 g fat (5 g saturated), 98 mg cholesterol, 95 mg sodium, 8 g total carbohydrates (5 g sugars), 1 g fiber, 36 g protein

Raspberry-Pistachio Crusted Chicken

Raspberries are filled with disease-preventing nutrients, and pistachios add color and flavor to a waist-friendly skinless chicken breast—yet another delicious way to get the lean protein necessary for maintaining a normal weight. Serve this over a bed of steamed shredded kale to up the nutrient factor even further.

½	cup raspberries
1	teaspoon Dijon mustard
1	tablespoon fresh lemon juice
¼	cup whole grain breadcrumbs (about ½ slice)
1	tablespoon coarsely ground pistachio nuts
1	tablespoon minced parsley
1	Dash of ground white pepper
1	Pinch of sea salt
2	skinless, boneless chicken breast halves
1	teaspoon olive oil

Combine raspberries, mustard, and lemon juice in a food processor or blender and process until smooth. Transfer to a shallow bowl or pie plate.

In another bowl, combine breadcrumbs, pistachios, parsley, pepper, and salt.

Place the chicken breasts between 2 pieces of wax paper and pound with the flat side of a meat pounder or a small heavy skillet to a ½-inch thickness. Dip chicken into the raspberry sauce, then into the breadcrumb mixture to coat.

Heat the oil in a skillet over medium heat. Add chicken cook until opaque throughout but still juicy, about 5 minutes per side. Serve each chicken breast on a bed of kale.

Serves 2

Per serving: 264 calories, 7 g fat (1 g saturated), 66 mg cholesterol, 408 mg sodium, 20 g total carbohydrates (2 g sugars), 5 g fiber, 32 g protein

Poached Halibut in Vegetable Broth

Maintaining a healthy weight is important for good sleep, as being over-weight increases the risk of snoring, obstructive sleep apnea, and back pain. Poached halibut is low in calories and high in omega-3 fatty acids—a perfect light yet satisfying meal.

4	skinless fillets (4 ounces each) halibut
2	cups slivered snow peas
1	cup bean sprouts
2	red bell peppers, cut into thin slivers
1	red onion, cut into thin slivers
1	cup carrot matchsticks
¼	cup minced garlic (about 10 cloves)
1	tablespoon finely chopped fresh ginger
1	teaspoon grated lemon zest
3	cups vegetable broth
1	cup sherry (optional)
3	tablespoons chopped cilantro

Put all the ingredients except cilantro into a large skillet with a lid. Bring to a simmer over high heat. Reduce the heat to low, cover, and cook until the halibut is just cooked through, about 6 minutes. Uncover, add cilantro, and cook for 2 minutes longer.

Serves 4

Per serving: 214 calories, 3 g fat (0.5 g saturated), 36 mg cholesterol, 362 mg sodium, 19 g total carbohydrates (8 g sugars), 1 g fiber, 27 g protein

Glazed Halibut
with Broccoli and Oranges

There's no question that fish is an important part of a balanced diet. The glazed halibut with broccoli and oranges will tempt your taste buds as it provides you with the necessary omega-3 fatty acids for good health.

1	pound red onions (about 4 medium)
3	teaspoons canola oil
¼	teaspoon salt
2	navel oranges
4	skinless halibut fillets or steaks (about 3 ounces each)
1	tablespoon honey
4	cups broccoli florets
	Freshly ground black pepper

Preheat the oven to 375°F. Line a large rimmed baking sheet with foil. Coat the foil with cooking spray.

Halve the onions crosswise and place, cut sides down, on a work surface. Cut into ½-inch-thick slices. Break the slices into separate pieces and transfer to the baking sheet. Drizzle with 2 teaspoons of the oil and ⅛ teaspoon of the salt. Toss to coat. Spread the onions in a single layer and roast, turning occasionally, until golden, about 20 minutes.

Meanwhile, grate 2 teaspoons zest from 1 orange. Peel and segment both oranges. When the onions are golden brown, add the orange segments and toss to coat. Return to the oven for 5 minutes.

Remove the baking sheet from the oven. Spread the onion and orange mixture into a single layer and lay the halibut on top. Drizzle the honey and ½ teaspoon of the reserved orange zest over the halibut. Return to the oven until the halibut is opaque, about 10 minutes.

Meanwhile, bring the remaining 1 teaspoon oil and 2 tablespoons water to a boil in a nonstick skillet. Add the broccoli and remaining ⅛ teaspoon salt. Cover and cook, tossing occasionally, until the broccoli is bright green and still crisp, about 5 minutes. Add the remaining orange zest and toss.

Divide the onion mixture among 4 plates and lay the fish on top. Serve with the broccoli, seasoning to taste with pepper at the table.

Serves 4

Per serving: 239 calories, 6 g fat (1 g saturated), 27 mg cholesterol, 216 mg sodium, 27 g total carbohydrates (15 g sugars), 6 g fiber, 22 g protein

Roasted Salmon with Mustard-Dill Glaze

Cut dinner preparation time in half with this simple salmon dish. Salmon is high in protein, low in calories, and a perfect way to add more fish into your meal plan. Complement the salmon with a fresh green salad and brown rice or whole grain bread for added good carbs.

3	tablespoons mayonnaise
1	tablespoon grainy mustard
1	tablespoon chopped fresh dill
1½	teaspoons dark brown sugar
1	teaspoon fresh lemon juice
4	center-cut salmon fillets (4 ounces each)
½	teaspoon salt
⅛	teaspoon ground black pepper

Preheat the oven to 400°F. Line a baking sheet with foil.

Combine the mayonnaise, mustard, dill, brown sugar, and lemon juice in a small bowl. Place the salmon on the baking sheet and season with the salt and pepper. Spread the mayonnaise mixture on top of the fillets and roast for 12 to 15 minutes, or until just cooked through.

Serves 4

Per serving: 298 calories, 21 g fat (3.5 g saturated), 71 mg cholesterol, 444 mg sodium, 4 g total carbohydrates (3 g sugars), 0 g fiber, 23 g protein

Shrimp Pasta Primavera

You can wait until the last guests arrive for dinner to prepare the shrimp pasta primavera. The pasta, shrimp, and vegetables are all cooked together in a pot of boiling water. In just minutes, you will have a filling meal that is high in protein and low in calories.

8	ounces whole grain penne pasta
1	pound frozen medium shrimp, thawed, peeled, and deveined
1	bag (16 ounces) frozen broccoli, onions, mushrooms, and peppers
½	cup fat-free plain Greek yogurt
¼	cup low-fat Caesar salad dressing
2	tablespoons shredded Parmesan cheese

Bring a medium pot of water to a boil. Cook the pasta according to package directions or until al dente, adding the shrimp and vegetables during the last 3 minutes of cooking. Drain well.

Meanwhile, whisk together the yogurt and salad dressing in a large bowl. Add the hot pasta and vegetables and toss to coat well. Sprinkle with the cheese.

Serves 4

Per serving: 417 calories, 5 g fat (1 g saturated), 176 mg cholesterol, 421 mg sodium, 54 g total carbohydrates (7 g sugars), 6.5 g fiber, 34 g protein

Salmon with Wild Rice Salad

Spinach, pine nuts, and celery add a flavorful surprise when served over the wild salmon fillets. Low in calories and high in omega-3 fatty acids, salmon is an easy way to add more fish to your meal plan.

1	**cup wild rice**
4	**cups chopped spinach**
2	**ribs celery, sliced**
1	**beet, peeled and shredded**
3	**tablespoons balsamic vinegar**
2	**tablespoons olive oil**
4	**teaspoons pine nuts**
¼	**teaspoon ground black pepper**
¾	**teaspoon salt**
4	**wild salmon fillets (4 ounces each)**

Cook the wild rice according to package directions.

Meanwhile, combine the spinach, celery, beet, vinegar, oil, pine nuts, pepper, and ½ teaspoon of the salt in a large bowl.

When the rice is done, drain if necessary, then add it to the vegetables and stir to combine.

Coat a large nonstick skillet with cooking spray and heat over medium heat. Add the salmon and cook, turning once, until the fish is opaque, about 6 minutes. Sprinkle with the remaining ¼ teaspoon salt.

Divide the fish and salad among 4 plates.

Serves 4

Per serving: 416 calories, 17 g fat (2.5 g saturated), 63 mg cholesterol, 575 mg sodium, 38 g total carbohydrates (5 g sugars), 5 g fiber, 30 g protein

Pasta Shells with Broccoli, Chickpeas, and Tomatoes

Eating a light meal at night is important to feeling relaxed for good sleep. This meatless dish is rich in flavor and complex carbohydrates—important for feeling calm and drowsy at bedtime.

2	cups pasta shells
	Salt
1	bag (14 ounces) frozen cut broccoli
1	tablespoon extra-virgin olive oil
1	can (15.5 ounces) chickpeas, rinsed and drained
1	clove garlic, crushed through a press or grated
1	teaspoon dried oregano
1/8	teaspoon red pepper flakes
1	can (14.5 ounces) diced tomatoes
1/4	cup grated pecorino Romano or Parmesan cheese

Bring a large pot of water to a boil. Add the pasta and salt to taste. Cook the pasta according to package directions or until al dente, adding the broccoli for the last 2 minutes of cooking. Ladle out and reserve ⅔ cup cooking liquid. Drain the pasta and broccoli and return to the pot.

Meanwhile, heat the oil in a 10-inch skillet over medium-high heat. Add the chickpeas, garlic, oregano, and red pepper flakes and cook, stirring gently, until the chickpeas turn golden in spots, about 3 minutes. Stir in the tomatoes (with juice), cover, and cook for 5 minutes over low heat to blend the flavors.

Stir the chickpea mixture and the reserved pasta cooking water into the drained pasta-broccoli mixture.

Serve in bowls and top with the cheese.

Serves 4

Per serving: 376 calories, 7 g fat (1.5 g saturated), 4.5 mg cholesterol, 398 mg sodium, 64.5 g total carbohydrates (6 g sugars), 10 g fiber, 16 g protein

Black Sesame Tofu and Vegetable Stir-Fry

Choosing nighttime meals that are light and high in complex carbohydrates is important for good sleep. This tofu and vegetable stir-fry is packed with the necessary nutrients you need to feel relaxed and drowsy at bedtime.

1	package (14 ounces) extra-firm tofu
1	teaspoon toasted sesame oil
2	tablespoons peanut oil
1½	tablespoons black sesame seeds
3	tablespoons fresh orange juice
2	tablespoons white miso
1	tablespoon reduced-sodium soy sauce
½	teaspoon cornstarch
1	pound asparagus, cut into 2-inch pieces
2	cups shredded carrots (about 6 ounces)
1	large yellow or red bell pepper, cut into thin strips
4	scallions, cut crosswise into 1-inch lengths
1⅓	cups cooked brown rice

Place the tofu on a plate and put a second plate on top. Weight the plate with one or two heavy cans and set aside for 10 to 15 minutes to press out some of the liquid. Cut crosswise into 8 slices.

Heat the sesame oil and 1 tablespoon of the peanut oil in a large nonstick skillet over medium-high heat. Place the sesame seeds in a shallow bowl and dredge the tofu slices in the seeds. Fry the tofu slices in the oil until nicely browned on one side, 4 to 5 minutes. Flip over and cook until nicely browned on the second side, 4 to 5 minutes. Transfer the tofu to a paper towel–lined plate.

Combine the orange juice, miso, soy sauce, and cornstarch in a small bowl. Whisk until well blended and set aside.

Heat the remaining 1 tablespoon peanut oil in the skillet. Stir in the asparagus and carrots and stir-fry until crisp-tender, about 4 minutes. Stir in the bell pepper and scallions and cook for 2 minutes. Reduce the heat to low and return the tofu to the pan. Pour the orange-miso mixture into the skillet and cook for 1 minute, stirring to coat the vegetables and tofu.

Serve over the rice.

Serves 4

Per serving: 359 calories, 17 g fat (2.5 g saturated), 0 mg cholesterol, 558 mg sodium, 38 g total carbohydrates (9.5 g sugars), 8.5 g fiber, 18 g protein

Quinoa Stir-Fry
with Spinach and Walnuts

The delectable combination of flavors in the quinoa stir-fry will calm your mood after a busy day. Walnuts and Parmesan cheese add protein to a dish that is naturally high in calming complex carbohydrates.

1	cup quinoa
2	tablespoons extra-virgin olive oil
1	teaspoon minced garlic
½	teaspoon salt
2	cups of water
½	cup walnut pieces
1	bag (6 ounces) baby spinach
1	cup grape or cherry tomatoes
½	cup grated Parmigiano-Reggiano cheese
	Torn fresh basil leaves, for garnish

Combine the quinoa and water to cover in a small bowl. Swish to rinse. Pour into a fine-mesh strainer and drain well.

Heat the oil in a medium skillet. Add the quinoa and toast, stirring, over medium heat until golden, about 10 minutes. Add the garlic and cook, stirring, for 1 minute. Add the salt and 2 cups water. Bring to a boil, reduce the heat to medium-low, cover, and cook until the water is absorbed, about 15 minutes.

Meanwhile, stir the walnuts in a small skillet over medium-low heat until toasted, about 5 minutes. Set aside.

When the quinoa is cooked, add the spinach and tomatoes to the skillet. Cook, stirring, over medium heat until the spinach is almost wilted and the tomatoes are warmed, about 1 minute. Stir in the toasted walnuts and cheese. Serve warm, garnished with basil.

Serves 4

Per serving: 396 calories, 22 g fat (3.5 g saturated), 9 mg cholesterol, 528 mg sodium, 37 g total carbohydrates (3 g sugars), 14 g fiber, 14 g protein

Miso Noodle Bowl

The miso noodle bowl is an all-time favorite that doesn't require a lot of effort. Flavorful and filling, this pasta dish is high in good carbs that will help calm you down with a serotonin buzz.

4	ounces whole wheat angel-hair pasta
2	cups vegetable or chicken broth
1	teaspoon ground ginger
3	cups water
2	carrots, thinly sliced on the diagonal
1	head broccoli (about 1 pound), cut into florets
¼	cup miso (any flavor)
16	ounces firm tofu, cut into ¼-inch cubes
4	scallions, sliced
1	tablespoon toasted sesame oil

Bring a medium pot of water to a boil. Add the pasta and cook according to package directions. Drain.

Meanwhile, combine the broth, ginger, and 3 cups water in a large saucepot or Dutch oven and bring to a boil over high heat. Add the carrots and broccoli and return to a boil. Reduce the heat to low, cover, and simmer until the vegetables are crisp-tender, about 5 minutes.

Place the miso in a small bowl and whisk in about 3 tablespoons of the hot broth from the saucepot. Then pour the miso back into the pot.

Stir in the drained pasta, tofu, scallions, and sesame oil and simmer for 3 minutes or until heated through.

Serves 4

Per serving: 310 calories, 8.5 g fat (1 g saturated), 0 mg cholesterol, 782 mg sodium, 48 g total carbohydrates (11 g sugars), 10 g fiber, 16 g protein

Roasted Squash and Shiitakes

Looking for the ultimate comfort food? Then say yes to the roasted squash and shiitakes. This easy recipe is high in flavor and complex carbohydrates and low in fat and calories.

⅓	cup sun-dried tomatoes
3	tablespoons olive oil
6	cloves garlic, sliced
6	cups cubed (1-inch) butternut squash
½	pound fresh shiitake mushrooms, stems discarded, caps thickly sliced
2	large Braeburn or other juicy red apples, unpeeled, cut into 1-inch chunks
1	teaspoon dried rosemary leaves, crumbled
½	teaspoon salt
¼	cup grated Parmesan cheese

Combine the sun-dried tomatoes and boiling water to cover in a small heatproof bowl. Let sit for 20 minutes to soften. Drain, reserving the liquid, and cut the tomatoes in thin slivers.

Preheat the oven to 400°F.

Combine the oil and garlic in a large roasting pan. Heat for 3 minutes in the oven. Add the sun-dried tomatoes and their soaking liquid, the squash, mushrooms, apples, rosemary, and salt, and toss to combine. Roast for 30 minutes, tossing the vegetables every 10 minutes, until tender. Sprinkle the Parmesan on top and roast for 5 minutes longer.

Serves 4

Per serving: 300 calories, 12 g fat (2.5 g saturated), 5 mg cholesterol, 476 mg sodium, 47 g total carbohydrates (19 g sugars), 8.5 g fiber, 7 g protein

Brown Rice Pilaf
with Apricots and Almonds

Need a side dish to complement fish or poultry? Try this fruit- and nut-studded pilaf. The unique combination of whole grain brown rice and fruity apricots not only tastes good—it's good for you too.

1¾	cups reduced-sodium chicken broth
¾	teaspoon salt
1¾	cups + 2 tablespoons water
1¾	cups medium-grain brown rice
1	tablespoon olive oil
1	cup finely chopped Vidalia or other sweet onion
¼	cup chopped dried apricots
2	teaspoons grated lemon peel
¼	teaspoon ground black pepper
2	tablespoons chopped fresh parsley
¼	cup slivered almonds

Combine the broth, salt, and 1¾ cups water in a saucepan. Bring to a boil, add the rice, reduce the heat to low, cover, and cook for 40 minutes. Remove from the heat and let stand, covered, for 5 minutes.

Ten minutes before the rice is finished, heat the oil in a skillet over medium-low heat. Add the onion and cook, stirring, until just soft, about 5 minutes. Add the apricots, lemon peel, pepper, and 2 tablespoons water. Stir well and remove from the heat.

Once the rice is done, uncover and toss with the onion mixture, parsley, and almonds.

Serves 8

Per serving: 212 calories, 5 g fat (1 g saturated), 0 mg cholesterol, 240 mg sodium, 38 g total carbohydrates (3.5 g sugars), 3 g fiber, 5 g protein

Buckwheat and Red Lentil Pilaf

Here's a versatile dish to replace plain rice or potatoes. Buckwheat groats—delicately flavored with apples, raisins, walnuts, and lentils—are a delicious and interesting way to bring more complex carbs to your dinner plate.

¼	cup walnut halves
2	teaspoons olive oil
4	cloves garlic, minced
1	cup roasted buckwheat groats (kasha)
½	cup red lentils
2	cups boiling water
1	cup carrot juice
¾	teaspoon ground coriander
¾	teaspoon salt
½	teaspoon ground black pepper
½	cup raisins
1	Granny Smith apple, peeled and diced
2	teaspoons walnut oil or olive oil

Toast the walnuts in a 350°F toaster oven or small ungreased skillet over medium heat until crisp and fragrant, 5 to 7 minutes. When cool enough to handle, coarsely chop. Heat the oil in a large skillet over medium heat. Add the garlic and cook until softened, about 1 minute. Stir in the buckwheat groats and lentils, and cook until the buckwheat is well coated, about 3 minutes. Add the boiling water, carrot juice, coriander, salt, and pepper, and bring to a boil. Reduce to a simmer, cover, and cook until the buckwheat is tender, about 15 minutes.

Stir in the toasted walnuts, raisins, apple, and walnut oil.

Serves 6

Per serving: 276 calories, 7 g fat (1 g saturated), 0 mg cholesterol, 311 mg sodium, 49 g total carbohydrates (12 g sugars), 9.5 g fiber, 9 g protein

Desserts

Blueberry Cheesecake Parfaits

If cheesecake is your guilty pleasure, you'll love this parfait. Not only do you get the serotonin boost from its high carb content, you also benefit from an added dose of disease-preventing antioxidants. Blueberries are super fruits that are also super soothers when it comes to sleep readiness.

4	ounces Neufchâtel cheese, at room temperature
½	cup reduced-fat sour cream
¼	cup confectioners' sugar
1	tablespoon pure vanilla extract
4	gingersnaps, crushed (2 to 3 tablespoons)
1½	cups fresh or thawed frozen blueberries

Combine the Neufchâtel and sour cream in a bowl and beat with an electric mixer on high speed until smooth. Add sugar and vanilla and beat until well combined. Measure out 4 teaspoons of the mixture and set aside. (You should have 1 cup for the parfaits.)

Fill each of 4 small parfait glasses or champagne flutes with layers, starting with 2 tablespoons of the cheese mixture, then some cookie crumbs, and then a layer of blueberries. Repeat the pattern once more using the remaining cheese mixture, crumbs, and blueberries. Finish by dabbing 1 teaspoon of the reserved cheese mixture on top of each parfait. Use any extra berries and crumbs to garnish, if desired. Chill at least 30 minutes before serving.

Serves 4

Per serving: 203 calories, 10 g fat (6 g saturated), 31 mg cholesterol, 189 mg sodium, 24 g total carbohydrates (15 g sugars), 1.5 g fiber, 5 g protein

Strawberry-Yogurt Shortcakes

Tired of smoothies? Yogurt and berries, a classic combination that also boast ample protein and carbs for welcoming sleep, are the filling for these lightened-up lower-fat biscuits.

2	cups low-fat vanilla yogurt
2	cups whole wheat pastry flour
4	tablespoons chilled butter, cut into small pieces
2	tablespoons packed light brown sugar
2	teaspoons baking powder
¼	teaspoon baking soda
⅔	cup plus 1 tablespoon low-fat buttermilk
1	tablespoon plus ⅓ cup granulated sugar
2	pints strawberries, sliced
3	tablespoons orange juice
1	teaspoon grated orange zest

Line a sieve with a coffee filter or white paper towel and place over a deep bowl. Place the yogurt in the sieve. Cover with plastic wrap, refrigerate, and allow to drain for 4 hours, or until very thick. Discard the liquid in the bowl.

Preheat the oven to 400°F. Coat a large baking sheet with cooking spray.

In a large bowl, combine the flour, butter, brown sugar, baking powder, and baking soda. Mix with your fingers to form crumbs. Add ⅔ cup of the buttermilk, stirring with a fork until the dough comes together. Turn the dough out onto a lightly floured surface. Gently pat or roll to a ¾-inch thickness. Using a 3-inch round cutter or large glass, cut into 6 biscuits. (You may have to pat the dough scraps together to cut out all the biscuits.) Place on the baking sheet. Brush with the remaining 1 tablespoon buttermilk and sprinkle with 1 tablespoon of the granulated sugar.

Bake until golden, about 12 minutes. Cool on the sheet on a rack for 10 minutes, then transfer to the rack to cool completely.

Combine the strawberries, orange juice, and the remaining ⅓ cup granulated sugar in a large bowl and toss well. Let stand for 10 minutes, stirring occasionally.

Whisk together the drained yogurt and orange zest in a medium bowl. Split the biscuits in half horizontally. On dessert plates, layer the biscuits with berries in the center and on the top. Top with the yogurt.

Serves 6

Per serving: 367 calories, 10 g fat (6 g saturated), 25 mg cholesterol, 328 mg sodium, 63 g total carbohydrates (36 g sugars), 5 g fiber, 10 g protein

Peachy Frozen Yogurt

You will feel relaxed and carefree after indulging in this light peachy frozen yogurt. It takes just minutes to whip up, and about 10 hours for the yogurt fruit mixture to freeze before eating.

3	**cups frozen peaches or nectarines, partially thawed**
1	**container (32 ounces) low-fat vanilla yogurt**
¼	**cup honey**

Place 1½ cups of the peaches in a food processor with the yogurt and honey. Process until smooth. Finely chop the remaining peaches and stir into the yogurt mixture. Pour into a 2-quart pan. Cover and freeze for 4 hours, or until firm.

Break the frozen mixture into small pieces and place in a food processor. Pulse until fluffy. Return the mixture to the pan and freeze, covered, for 6 hours, or until firm. Let the frozen yogurt stand at room temperature for 15 minutes before serving.

Serves 12

Per serving: 98 calories, 1 g fat (0.5 g saturated), 4 mg cholesterol, 50 mg sodium, 20 g total carbohydrates (19 g sugars), 0.5 g fiber, 4 g protein

Raspberry Peaches with Greek Yogurt

Want a rich-tasting bedtime snack without a guilt trip? This fits the bill perfectly. The thick, tart yogurt is packed with calcium and the right balance of carbohydrate and protein to calm you down before bed.

1	**medium peach, chopped**
1	**tablespoon raspberry spreadable fruit**
1	**teaspoon orange juice or water**
	Pinch of apple pie spice
1	**cup fat-free plain Greek yogurt**

Combine the peach, spreadable fruit, orange juice or water, and apple pie spice in a medium bowl and stir gently to combine. Using a slotted spoon, spoon just the peaches into a dessert bowl. Top with the yogurt and drizzle with the raspberry juices.

Serves 1

Per serving: 223 calories, 1 g fat (0 g saturated), 0 mg cholesterol, 83 mg sodium, 35 g total carbohydrates (31 g sugars), 2 g fiber, 20 g protein

Frozen Banana Yogurt Pops

Make these ahead of time, so they are always on hand, then pull out a frozen pop as a bedtime snack when you need melt-in-your-mouth goodness. At fewer than 200 calories each, the frozen pops have the perfect ratio of carbs to protein to ensure a good night's sleep.

3	cups fat-free plain Greek yogurt
2	cups frozen unsweetened strawberries
1	medium banana
2	teaspoons pure vanilla extract
2	tablespoons agave nectar or honey

Combine the yogurt, strawberries, banana, vanilla extract, and nectar or honey in a blender. Process until smooth. Pour the mixture into 4 ice-pop molds or paper cups. Place an ice-pop stick in the middle of each cup and freeze for 2 hours, or until solid. To serve, remove from the molds or peel away the paper cups.

Serves 4

Per serving: 178 calories, 0 g fat (0 g saturated), 0 mg cholesterol, 64 mg sodium, 29 g total carbohydrates (22 g sugars), 2 g fiber, 15 g protein

Notes

Chapter 1: The Sleep/Weight Connection

1   Altemus, M., B. Rao, F. Dhabha, et al. Stress-induced changes in skin barrier function in healthy women. *Journal of Investigative Dermatology* 2001;117:309–17.

2   *British Medical Journal,* www.bmj.com/content/341/bmj.c6614.full.pdf-html.

3   National Sleep Foundation. Women and sleep. n.d. http://www.sleepfoundation.org/article/sleep-topics/women-and-sleep.

4   Vgontzas, A.N., E. Zoumakis, E.O. Bixler, et al. Adverse effects of modest sleep restriction on sleepiness, performance, and inflammatory cytokines. *Journal of Clinical Endocrinology and Metabolism* 2004;89:2119–26.

5   National Sleep Foundation. 2005 *Sleep in America* poll: Summary of findings. Washington, DC: National Sleep Foundation, 2005.

6   National Center for Health Statistics. QuickStats: Percentage of adults who reported an average of ≤6 hours of sleep per 24-hour period, by sex and age group—United States, 1985 and 2004. *Morbidity and Mortality Weekly Report* 2005;54:933.

7   Patel, S.R., F.B. Hu. Short sleep duration and weight gain: A systematic review. *Obesity (Silver Spring)* 2008;3:643–53.

8   Watanabe, M., H. Kikuchi, K. Tanaka, M. Takahashi. Association of short sleep duration with weight gain and obesity at 1-year follow-up: A large-scale prospective study. *Sleep* 2010;33:161–67.

9   National Center for Health Statistics. Prevalence of overweight, obesity and extreme obesity among adults: United States, trends 1976–1980 through 2005–2006. *Health E-Stat,* December 2008. http://www.cdc.gov/nchs/data/hestat/overweight/overweight_adult.pdf.

10 National Sleep Foundation. How much sleep do we really need? n.d. http://www.sleepfoundation.org/article/how-sleep-works/how-much-sleep-do-we-really-need.

11 Ibid.

12 Institute of Medicine. *Sleep disorders and sleep deprivation: An unmet public health problem.* Washington, DC: National Academies Press, 2006.

13 Mokdad, A., B. Bowman, E. Ford, et al. The continuing epidemics of obesity and diabetes in the United States. *JAMA* 2001;286:1195–1200.

14 Knutson, K.L., K. Spiegel, P. Penev, E. Van Cauter. The metabolic consequences of sleep deprivation. *Sleep Medicine Reviews* 2007;11(3):163–78.

15 Golden, L., H. Jorgensen. Time after time: Mandatory overtime in the U.S. economy. Economic Policy Institute Briefing Paper #120, January 1, 2002. http://www.epi.org/publications/entry/briefingpapers_bp120.

16 Williams, J.C., H. Boushey, The three faces of work-family conflict. Center for American Progress, January 25, 2010. http://www.americanprogress.org/issues/2010/01/three_faces_report.html.

17   National Institute of Mental Health. Anxiety disorders. n.d. http://www.nimh.nih.gov/health/topics/anxiety-disorders/index.shtml.

18   Anxiety Disorders Association of America. Facts and statistics. n.d. http://www.adaa.org/about-adaa/press-room/facts-statistics.

19   National Institute of Mental Health. *Anxiety disorders.* NIH Publication No. 09-3879, 2009. http://www.nimh.nih.gov/health/publications/anxiety-disorders/complete-index.shtml.

20   Wilson TV. How women work. HowStuffWorks.com. n.d. http://people.howstuffworks.com/women.htm.

21   Owens, J., R. Maxim, M. McGuinn, et al. Television-viewing habits and sleep disturbance in school children. *Pediatrics* 1999;104(3):e27.

22   Kantermann, T., T. Roenneberg. Is light-at-night a health risk factor or a health risk predictor? *Chronobiology International* 2009;26(6):1069–74.

23   Ibid.

24   Williams, J.C., H. Boushey. The three faces of work-family conflict. Center for American Progress, January 25, 2010. http://www.americanprogress.org/issues/2010/01/three_faces_report.html.

25   Patel, S.R., A. Malhotra, D.P. White, et al. Association between reduced sleep and weight gain in women. *American Journal of Epidemiology* 2006;164:947–54.

26   Gangwisch, J.E., D. Malaspina, B. Boden-Albala, et al. Inadequate sleep as a risk factor for obesity: Analyses of the NHANES I. *Sleep* 2005;28(10):1289–96.

27   National Sleep Foundation. 2009 *Sleep in America* poll: Summary of findings. Washington, DC: National Sleep Foundation, 2009. http://www.sleepfoundation.org/sites/default/files/2009%20Sleep%20in%20America%20SOF%20EMBARGOED.pdf.

28   Nedeltcheva, A.V., J.M. Kilkus, J. Imperial, et al. Sleep curtailment is accompanied by increased intake of calories from snacks. *American Journal of Clinical Nutrition* 2009;89:126–33.

29   Van Cauter, E., K.L. Knutson. Sleep and the epidemic of obesity in children and adults. *European Journal of Endocrinology* 2008;159 Suppl 1:S59–66.

30   Nedeltcheva, A.V., J.M. Kilkus, J. Imperial, et al. Sleep curtailment is accompanied by increased intake of calories from snacks. *American Journal of Clinical Nutrition* 2009;89(1):126–33.

31   Knutson, K.L. Impact of sleep and sleep loss on glucose homeostasis and appetite regulation. *Sleep Medicine Clinics* 2007;2(2):187–97.

32   Sanders, L. Lack of sleep has genetic link with type 2 diabetes: Large genomic studies show body rhythms, melatonin may influence sugar levels in the blood. *Science News* 2007;175:5, January 3.

33   Van Cauter, E., K.L. Knutson, P.J. Rathouz, et al. Association between sleep and blood pressure in midlife: The CARDIA sleep study. *Archives of Internal Medicine* 2009;169:1055–61.

34   Antunes, L.C., R. Levandovski, G. Dantas, et al. Obesity and shift work. *Nutrition Research Reviews* 2010;23(1):155–68.

35   Garaulet, M., J.A. Madrid, Chronobiology, genetics, and metabolic syndrome. *Current Opinion in Lipidology* 2009;20(2):127–34.

36   Katayose, Y., M. Tasaki, H. Ogata, et al. Metabolic rate and fuel utilization during sleep assessed by whole-body indirect calorimetry. *Metabolism: Clinical and Experimental* 2009;58(7):920–26.

37   Sivak, M. Sleeping more as a way to lose weight. *Obesity Reviews* 2006;7:295–96.

38 Ferber, R. *How to solve your child's sleep problems*. New York: Simon and Schuster, 1985.

39 National Center for Health Statistics. QuickStats: Percentage of adults who reported an average of ≤6 hours of sleep per 24-hour period, by sex and age group—United States, 1985 and 2004. *Morbidity and Mortality Weekly Report* 2005;54:933.

40 Redline, S., P. Elbert, P.E. Wright. The association of sleep duration with adolescents' fat and carbohydrate consumption. *Sleep* 33(9):1201–9.

41 National Sleep Foundation. Teens and sleep. n.d. http://www.sleepfoundation.org/article/sleep-topics/teens-and-sleep.

Chapter 2: What Happens While You Sleep?

1 Borbely, A.A. A two process model of sleep regulation. *Human Neurobiology* 1982;1(3):195–204.

2 Breus, M.J. Skin cells and circadian rhythms. Sleep Well, WebMD.com, February 21, 2008. http://blogs.webmd.com/sleep-disorders/2008/02/skin-cells-and-circadian-rhythms.html.

3 Thomson, E.A. Rest easy: MIT study confirms melatonin's value as sleep aid. MIT News, March 1, 2005. http://web.mit.edu/newsoffice/2005/melatonin.html.

4 Martin, S.E., H.M. Engleman, I.J. Deary, N.J. Douglas. The effect of sleep fragmentation on daytime function. *American Journal of Respiratory and Critical Care Medicine* 1996;153:1328–32.

5 National Women's Health Information Center. Insomnia: Do more women than men have insomnia? February 17, 2010. http://www.womenshealth.gov/faq/Insomnia.cfm#c.

6 National Heart, Lung, and Blood Institute. Diseases and conditions index: Sleep apnea: Who is at risk for sleep apnea? August 2010. http://www.nhlbi.nih.gov/health/dci/Diseases/SleepApnea/SleepApnea_WhoIsAtRisk.html.

7 National Heart, Lung, and Blood Institute. Diseases and conditions index: Restless legs syndrome: Who is at risk for restless legs syndrome? November 2010. http://www.nhlbi.nih.gov/health/dci/Diseases/rls/rls_WhoIsAtRisk.html.

8 National Heart, Lung, and Blood Institute. Diseases and conditions index: Restless legs syndrome: Key points. November 2010. http://www.nhlbi.nih.gov/health/dci/Diseases/rls/rls_Summary.html.

9 Hirshkowitz, M., C.A. Moore, C.R. Hamilton, et al. Polysomnography of adults and elderly: Sleep architecture, respiration and leg movement. *Journal of Clinical Neurophysiology* 1992;9:56–62.

10 National Heart, Lung, and Blood Institute. Diseases and conditions index: Sleep apnea: Who is at risk for sleep apnea? http://www.nhlbi.nih.gov/health/dci/Diseases/SleepApnea/SleepApnea_WhoIsAtRisk.html.

11 Bio-Medicine.com. New study in JCSM shows effective treatment for elderly insomniacs: PLMS common in older women. October 1, 2006. http://news.bio-medicine.org/medicine-news-3/New-study-in-JCSM-shows-effective-treatment-for-elderly-insomniacs-2840-2.

Chapter 3: The Sleep/Metabolism Matrix

1 Turek, F.W., C. Joshu, A. Kohsaka, et al. Obesity and metabolic syndrome in circadian clock mutant mice. *Science* 2005;308:1043–45.

2 Stranges, S., F.P. Cappuccio, N.B. Kandala, et al. Cross-sectional versus prospective associations of sleep duration with changes in relative weight and body fat distribution: The Whitehall II study. *American Journal of Epidemiology* 2008;167(3):321–29.

3   Singh, M., C.L. Drake, T. Roehrs, et al. The association between obesity and short sleep duration: A population-based study. *Journal of Clinical Sleep Medicine* 2005;1:357–63.

4   Taheri, S., L. Lin, D. Austin, et al. Short sleep duration is associated with reduced leptin, elevated ghrelin, and increased body mass index. *PLoS Medicine* 1(3):e62. http://www.plosmedicine.org/article/info:doi/10.1371/journal.pmed.0010062#pmed-0010062-t002.

5   Katayose, Y., M. Tasaki, H. Ogata, et al. Metabolic rate and fuel utilization during sleep assessed by whole-body indirect calorimetry. *Metabolism: Clinical and Experimental* 58(7):920–26.

6   Nedeltcheva, A.V., J.M. Kilkus, J. Imperial, et al. Insufficient sleep undermines dietary efforts to reduce adiposity. *Annals of Internal Medicine* 2010;153(7):435–41.

7   American Diabetes Association. American Diabetes Association announces legislative priorities: Agenda for 2011 aimed at stopping diabetes. January 6, 2011. http://www.diabetes.org/for-media/2011/2011-legislative-priorities.html. [press release]

8   American Diabetes Association. Living with diabetes: Hypoglycemia (low blood glucose). n.d. http://www.diabetes.org/living-with-diabetes/treatment-and-care/blood-glucose-control/hypoglycemia-low-blood.html.

9   Knutson, K.L., K. Spiegel, P. Penev, E . Van Cauter. The metabolic consequences of sleep deprivation. *Sleep Medicine Reviews* 2007;11(3):163–78.

10 Spiegel, K., E. Tasali, P. Penev, E. Van Cauter. Sleep curtailment in healthy young men is associated with decreased leptin levels, elevated ghrelin levels, and increased hunger and appetite. *Annals of Internal Medicine* 2004;141:846–50.

11 Ibid.

12 Ibid.

13 Wang, J., A. Akabayashi, J. Dourmashkin, et al. Neuropeptide Y in relation to carbohydrate intake, corticosterone and dietary obesity. *Brain Research* 1998;802(1–2):75–88.

14 Epel, E.S., B. McEwen, T. Seeman, et al. Stress and body shape: Stress-induced cortisol secretion is consistently greater among women with central fat. *Psychosomatic Medicine* 2000;62(5):623–32.

15 Grossi, G., A. Perski, B. Evengard, et al. Physiological correlates of burnout among women. Journal of *Psychosomatic Research* 2003;55(4):309–16.

16 Tchernof, A., A. Nolan, C.K. Sites, et al. Weight loss reduces C-reactive protein levels in obese postmenopausal women. *Circulation* 2002;105(5):564–69.

17 American Psychological Association. Stress in America. October 7, 2008. http://www.apa.org/news/press/releases/2008/10/stress-in-america.pdf.

18 Nedeltcheva, A.V., J.M.Kilkus, J.Imperial, et al. Sleep curtailment is accompanied by increased intake of calories from snacks. *American Journal of Clinical Nutrition* 2009;89(1):126–33.

19 Tang-Christensen, M., N. Vrang, S. Ortmann, et al. Central administration of ghrelin and agouti-related protein (83-132) increases food intake and decreases spontaneous locomotor activity in rats. *Endocrinology* 2004;145:4645–52.

20 Schmid, S.M., M. Hallschmid, K. Jauch-Chara, et al. Short-term sleep loss decreases physical activity under free living conditions but does not increase food intake under time-deprived laboratory conditions in healthy men. *American Journal of Clinical Nutrition* 2009;90:1476–82.

21 Briones, B., N. Adams, M. Strauss, et al. Relationship between sleepiness and general health status. *Sleep* 1996;19:583–88.

Chapter 4: The Unique Sleep Challenges of Women

1   National Sleep Foundation. Menopause and sleep. n.d. http://www.sleepfoundation.org/article/sleep-topics/menopause-and-sleep.

2   National Center on Sleep Disorders Research. Sleep, sex differences, and women's health. *2003 National Sleep Disorders Research Plan,* July 2003. http://www.nhlbi.nih.gov/health/prof/sleep/res_plan/section4/section4a.html.

3   Phillips, B., N.A. Collop, C. Drake, et al. Sleep disorders and medical conditions in women. *Journal of Women's Health (*Larchmont*)* 2008;17(7):1191–99.

4   Young, T., D. Rabago, A. Zgierska, et al. Objective and subjective sleep quality in premeno-pausal, perimenopausal, and postmenopausal women in the Wisconsin Sleep Cohort Study. *Sleep* 2003;6(6):667–72.

5   Ikehara, S., H. Iso, C. Date, et al. Association of sleep duration with mortality from cardio-vascular disease and other causes for Japanese men and women: The JACC study. *Sleep* 2009;32:295–301.

6   Coyne, M.D., C.M. Kesick, T.J. Doherty, et al. Circadian rhythm changes in core temperature over the menstrual cycle: Method for noninvasive monitoring. *American Journal of Physiology: Regulatory, Integrative and Comparative Physiology* 2000; 279:R1316–20.

7   Van Cauter, E., R. Leproult, D.J. Kupfer. Effects of gender and age on the levels and circa-dian rhythmicity of plasma cortisol. *Journal of Clinical Endocrinology and Metabolism* 1996;81:2468–73.

8   National Sleep Research Project. 40 facts about sleep you probably didn't know. n.d. http://www.abc.net.au/science/sleep/facts.htm.

9   Silber, B.Y., J.A. Schmitt. Effects of tryptophan loading on human cognition, mood and sleep. *Neuroscience and Biobehavioral Reviews* 2010;34(3):387–407.

10 National Sleep Foundation. 2007 *Sleep in America* poll: Women and sleep. n.d. http://www.sleepfoundation.org/sites/default/files/Summary_Of_Findings%20-%20FINAL.pdf.

11 Thys-Jacobs, S., P. Starkey, D. Bernstein, et al. Calcium carbonate and the premenstrual syndrome: Effects on premenstrual and menstrual symptoms. *American Journal of Obstet-rics and Gynecology* 1998;179(2):444–52.

12 Singleton, G. Premenstrual disorders in adolescent females—Integrative management *Aus-tralian Family Physician* 2007;36(8):629–30.

13 Mizuno, S., T. Mihara, T. Miyaoka, et al. CSF iron, ferritin and transferrin levels in restless legs syndrome. *Journal of Sleep Research* 2005;14(1):43–47.

14 Kwan, I., J.L. Onwude. Premenstrual syndrome. *Clinical Evidence (*Online*)* 2007 May 1;2007:0806.

15 Zukov, I., R. Ptácek, J. Raboch, et al. Premenstrual dysphoric disorder—Review of actual findings about mental disorders related to menstrual cycle and possibilities of their therapy. *Prague Medical Report* 2010;111(1):12–24.

16 Ibid.

17 Kwan, I., J.L. Onwude. Premenstrual syndrome. *Clinical Evidence (*Online*)* 2007 May 1;2007:0806.

18 Baker, F.C., T.L. Kahan, J. Trinder, I.M. Colrain. Sleep quality and the sleep electroen-cephalogram in women with severe premenstrual syndrome. *Sleep* 2007;30(10):1283–91.

19 National Women's Health Information Center. Premenstrual syndrome. May 18, 2010. http://womenshealth.gov/faq/premenstrual-syndrome.cfm.

20 National Sleep Foundation. Pregnancy and sleep. n.d. http://www.sleepfoundation.org/article/sleep-topics/pregnancy-and-sleep.

21 Ibid.

22 Gunderson, E., S.L. Rifas-Shiman, E. Oken, et al. Association of fewer hours of sleep at 6 months postpartum with substantial weight retention at 1 year postpartum. *American Journal of Epidemiology* 2008;167(2):178–87.

23 National Sleep Foundation. Stressed-out American women have no time for sleep. March 6, 2007. http://www.sleepfoundation.org/sites/default/files/Poll Release—FINAL.pdf. [press release]

24 National Women's Health Information Center. Depression during and after pregnancy. March 6, 2009. http://www.womenshealth.gov/faq/depression-pregnancy.cfm.

25 Kayumov, L., R. Casper, R. Hawa, et al. Blocking low-wavelength light prevents nocturnal melatonin suppression with no adverse effect on performance during simulated shift work. *Journal of Clinical Endocrinology and Metabolism* 2005;90(5):2755–61.

26 Bennett, S., M. Alpert, V. Kubulins, R. Hansler. Use of modified spectacles and light bulbs to block blue light at night may prevent postpartum depression. *Medical Hypotheses* 2009;73:251–53.

27 Morris, R.S. Could leptin be the next fertility medication? IVF1.com, June 18, 2008. http://www.ivf1.com/leptin.

28 Roth, T., T. Roehrs, R. Pies. Insomnia: Pathophysiology and implications for treatment. *Sleep Medicine Reviews* 2007;11(1):71–79.

29 National Sleep Foundation. Stressed-out American women have no time for sleep. March 6, 2007. http://www.sleepfoundation.org/sites/default/files/Poll Release—FINAL.pdf. [press release]

30 Mayo Clinic. Belly fat in women: How to keep it off. April 16, 2009. http://www.mayoclinic.com/health/belly-fat/WO00128.

31 Nelson, H.D., E. Haney, L. Humphrey, et al. Management of Menopause-Related Symptoms. Evidence Reports/Technology Assessments, No. 120. Rockville (MD): Agency for Healthcare Research and Quality (US); 2005 Mar. http://www.ncbi.nlm.nih.gov/books/NBK37767/

32 Hollander, L.E., E.W. Freeman, M.D. Sammel, et al. Sleep quality, estradiol levels, and behavioral factors in late reproductive age women. *Obstetrics and Gynecology* 2001;98(3:)391–97.

33 Shanafelt, T., D. Barton, A. Adjei, C. Loprinzi. Pathophysiology and treatment of hot flashes. *Mayo Clinic Proceedings* 2002;77:1207–18.

34 National Sleep Foundation. 2007 *Sleep in America* poll: Women and sleep. n.d. http://www.sleepfoundation.org/sites/default/files/Summary_Of_Findings%20-%20FINAL.pdf.

35 Ohayon, M.M. Severe hot flashes are associated with chronic insomnia. *Archives of Internal Medicine* 2006;166(12):1262–68.

36 Nowakowski, S., C.J. Meliska, L.F. Martinez, B.L. Parry. Sleep and menopause. *Current Neurology and Neuroscience Reports* 2009;9(2):165–72.

37 Dancey, D., P. Hanly, C. Soong, et al. Impact of menopause on the prevalence and severity of sleep apnea. *Chest* 2001;120:151–55.

38 Young, T., D. Rabago, A. Zgierska, et al. Objective and subjective sleep quality in premenopausal, perimenopausal, and postmenopausal women in the Wisconsin Sleep Cohort Study. *Sleep* 2003;26(6):667–72.

39 Raymann, R.J.E.M., E.J.W. Van Someren. Diminished capability to recognize the optimal temperature for sleep initiation may contribute to poor sleep in elderly people. *Sleep* 2008;31(9):1301–9.

40 Ibid.

41 Ibid.

42 Ibid.

43 Parmeggiani, P.L. Temperature regulation during sleep: A study in homeostasis. In Orem J, Barnes CD (eds). *Physiology in sleep*. New York: Academic Press, 1980. pp. 98–143.

44 National Sleep Foundation. 2007 *Sleep in America* poll: Women and sleep. n.d. http://www .sleepfoundation.org/sites/default/files/Summary_Of_Findings%20-%20FINAL.pdf

45 National Sleep Foundation. Menopause and sleep. n.d. http://www.sleepfoundation.org/ article/sleep-topics/menopause-and-sleep.

46 Murphy, P.J., S.S. Campbell. Sex hormones, sleep, and core body temperature in older post-menopausal women. *Sleep* 2007;30(12):1788–94.

47 Ibid.

48 Dancy, D.R., P.J. Hanly, C. Soong, et al. Impact of menopause on the prevalence and severity of sleep apnea. *Chest* 2001;120:151–155.

49 Ibid.

50 Young, T., P.E. Peppard, D.J. Gottlieb. Epidemiology of obstructive sleep apnea. *American Journal of Respiratory and Critical Care Medicine* 2002;165:1217–39.

Chapter 6: The 5 Simple Rules for Better Sleep

1 National Institute on Alcohol Abuse and Alcoholism. Alcohol and sleep. Alcohol Alert no. 41, July 1998. http://pubs.niaaa.nih.gov/publications/aa41.htm.

2 Dusek, J.A., H. Benson. Mind-body medicine: A model of the comparative clinical impact of the acute stress and relaxation responses. *Minnesota Medicine* 2009;92(5):47–50.

3 Newsweek. Relaxation: Ways to calm your mind. Newsweek.com, October 3, 2004. http:// www.newsweek.com/2004/10/03/relaxation-ways-to-calm-your-mind.html.

4 American Psychological Association. Stress in America: October 7, 2008. http://www.apa .org/news/press/releases/2008/10/stress-in-america pdf.

5 Ibid.

6 Saey, T.H. A gene for short sleep: Genetic variation reduces amount of shut-eye in some people and in experiments on mice and fruit flies. *Science News*, September 12, 2009. p. 11.

7 He, Y., C.R. Jones, N. Fujiki, et al. The transcriptional repressor DEC2 regulates sleep length in mammals. *Science* 2009;325(5942):866–70.

8 McCusker, R.R., B.A. Goldberger, E.J. Cone. Technical note: Caffeine content of energy drinks, carbonated sodas, and other beverages. *Journal of Analytical Toxicology* 2006;30(2):112–14.

9 National Sleep Foundation. Caffeine and sleep. n.d. http://www.sleepfoundation.org/article/ sleep-topics/caffeine-and-sleep.

10 National Sleep Foundation. 2005 *Sleep in America* poll: Summary of findings. http://www .sleepfoundation.org/sites/default/files/2005_summary_of_findings.pdf.

11 Johnson, E.O., T. Roehrs, T. Roth, N.Breslau. Epidemiology of alcohol and medication as aids to sleep in early adulthood. *Sleep* 1998;21(2):178–86.

12 Passos, G.S. Physical exercise can improve sleep quality of insomniac patients? Abstract 737, presented at the 22nd Associated Professional Sleep Societies Meeting, June 7–12, 2008, Baltimore.

13 Brigham and Women's Hospital. Dodging weight gain with vitamin D. October 13, 2010. http://www.brighamandwomens.org/Patients_Visitors/pcs/nutrition/services/healtheweightforwomen/special_topics/DodgingWeightGainWithVitaminD.aspx?subID=submenu10.

14 Murphy, P.K., C.L. Wagner. "Vitamin C and mood disorders among women: an integrative review." Journal of Midwifery & Women's Health. 2008 Sep–Oct; 53 (5): 440–46.

15 Miller, A.L. Epidemiology, etiology, and natural treatment of seasonal affective disorder. *Alternative Medicine Review* 2005;10(1):5–13.

16 Coiro, V., R. Volpi, C. Marchesi, A. De Ferri. Abnormal serotonergic control of prolactin and cortisol secretion in patients with seasonal affective disorder. *Psychoneuroendocrinology* 1993;18(8):551–56.

17 Shipowick, C.D., C.B. Moore, C. Corbett, R. Bindler. Vitamin D and depressive symptoms in women during the winter: A pilot study. *Applied Nursing Research* 2009;22(3):221–25.

18 Rosenthal, N.E. Light therapy: Theory and practice. *Primary Psychiatry* 1984;Sep/Oct:31.

19 Mayo Clinic. Light therapy: Why it's done. October 7, 2010. http://www.mayoclinic.com/health/light-therapy/MY00195/DSECTION=why%2Dits%2Ddone.

20 MedlinePlus. Muscle aches. May 2, 2009. http://www.nlm.nih.gov/medlineplus/ency/article/003178.htm.

21 Huijuan, Cao et al. (2009). Acupuncture for Treatment of Insomnia: A systematic Review of Randomized Controlled Trials. *Journal of Alternative and Complementary Medicine* Vol 15, issue 11, 1171–86.

22 Field, T. Massage therapy effects. *American Psychologist* 1998;53(12):1270–81.

23 Schmidt, B., S. Hanslmayr. Resting frontal EEG alpha-asymmetry predicts the evaluation of affective musical stimuli. *Neuroscience Letters* 2009;460(3):237–40.

24 Lai, H.L., M. Good. Music improves sleep quality in older adults. *Journal of Advanced Nursing* 2004;49(3):234–44.

25 de Niet, G., B. Tiemens, B. Lendemeijer, G. Hutschemaekers. Music-assisted relaxation to improve sleep quality: Meta analysis. *Journal of Advanced Nursing* 2009;65(7):1356–64.

26 Marquardt, C.J.G., L.L. Orr, M. Perugini. A pilot study of EEG entrainment as a sleep aid. Tools for Wellness, n.d. http://www.toolsforwellness.com/delta-sleep-research.html.

Chapter 7: Design the Right Environment

1 National Sleep Foundation. Snoring and sleep. n.d. http://www.sleepfoundation.org/article/sleep-related-problems/snoring-and-sleep.

2 National Heart Lung and Blood Institute. Diseases and conditions index: Sleep apnea. August 2010. http://www.nhlbi.nih.gov/health/dci/Diseases/SleepApnea/SleepApnea_WhatIs.html.

3 Dog tired? It could be your pooch. ScienceDaily, February 15, 2002. http://www.sciencedaily.com/releases/2002/02/020215070932.htm.

4 Blumenthal, M., A. Goldberg, J. Brinckmann. *Herbal Medicine: Expanded Commission E Monographs*. Newton, MA: Integrative Medicine Communications, 2000. pp. 226–29.

5 Ibid.

Chapter 8: Eat Right to Sleep Tight

1   Nedeltcheva, A.V., J.M. Kilkus, J. Imperial, et al. Insufficient sleep undermines dietary efforts to reduce adiposity. *Annals of Internal Medicine* 2010;153(7):435–41.

2   Ikeda, M. (2002). Amino acid production processes. *Adv. Biochem. Eng. Biotechnol.*79: 1–35.

3   Schaechter, J.D., R.J. Wurtman. (1990). Serotonin release varies with brain tryptophan levels. *Brain Res.*532 (1-2): 203–10.

4   http://www.medicalnewstoday.com/articles/163169.php

5   Thomson, E.A. Carbs are essential for effective dieting and good mood, Wurtman says. *MIT News,* February 20, 2004. [press release]

6   Caruso, I., P. Sarzi Puttini, M. Cazzola, V. Azzolini. Double-blind study of 5-hydroxytryptophan versus placebo in the treatment of primary fibromyalgia syndrome. *Journal of International Medical Research* 1990;18:201–9.

7   Afaghi, A., H. O'Connor, C.N. Chow. High-glycemic-index carbohydrate meals shorten sleep onset. *American Journal of Clinical Nutrition* 2007;85(2):426–30.

8   Fundukian, L.J., ed. *The Gale Encyclopedia of Alternative Medicine,* 3rd edition. Detroit: Gale, Cengage Learning, 2009.

9   Mooney, S., J.E. Leuendorf, C. Hendrickson, et al. Vitamin B_6: A long known compound of surprising complexity. *Molecules* 2009;14(1):329–51.

10 Honma, K., M. Kohsaka, N. Fukuda, et al. Effects of vitamin B_{12} on plasma melatonin rhythm in humans: Increased light sensitivity phase-advances the circadian clock? *Experientia* 48:716–20.

11 National Center for Complementary and Alternative Medicine. *Sleep disorders and CAM.* NCCAM Publication No. D437, September 2010. http://nccam.nih.gov/health/sleep/ataglance.htm.

12 University of Maryland Medical Center. Lavender. March 12, 2009. http://www.umm.edu/altmed/articles/lavender-000260.htm.

13 De Benedittis, G., R. Massei. Serotonin precursors in chronic primary headache: A double-blind cross-over study with L-5-hydroxytryptophan vs. placebo. *Journal of Neurosurgical Sciences* 1985;29:239–48.

14 National Center for Complementary and Alternative Medicine. *Herbs at a Glance: A Quick Guide to Herbal Supplements.* NIH Publication No. 10-6248, June 2010. http://nccam.nih.gov/health/NIH_Herbs_at_a_Glance.pdf.

15 Institute of Medicine, Food and Nutrition Board. *Dietary reference intakes for calcium and vitamin D.* Washington, DC: National Academies Press, 2010.

16 Pigeon, W.R., M. Carr, C. Gorman, M.L. Perlis. Effects of a tart cherry juice beverage on the sleep of older adults with insomnia: A pilot study. *Journal of Medicinal Food* 2010;13(3):579–83.

Index

Boldface page references indicate illustrations. Underscored references indicate boxed text.

A

Abdominal fat, 48
Acne, worsening with sleep loss, 8
Active state, sleep as, 26–27
Acupuncture, insomnia for, 121
ADHD, 10
Adrenal glands, 46, 47
Adrenaline
  decrease with relaxation response, 101
  increase with caffeine, 108
  release during stress or anxiety, 13, 47
Adrenocorticotropin, insomnia and, 70
Aerobic exercise, body temperature elevation
      from, 97, 113
Air filter, 163, 166–67
Air purifier, 163, 166–67
Air quality, 165–66
Alarm clocks, 153, 156–58
Alcohol
  avoidance before bedtime, 59, 97, 111–12
  blood alcohol level, 97
  PMS effect on blood level of, 59
  sleep apnea worsening from, 97
Alertness, decrease during PMS, 62
Almonds
  Brown Rice Pilaf with Apricots and
      Almonds, 223
Alpha waves, 101, 129, 163
Amino acids, 170
Anemia, during menstrual cycle, 60
Antihistamine, 172
Antioxidants
  in black tea, 110
  in red wine, 112
Anxiety
  beneficial aspects of, 13
  calming
    with foods that boost serotonin, 170,
      171

  with meditation, 126–28
  with music, 129–31
  with self-massage, 128–29
  disorders, 13
  increase with poor sleep, 10
  insomnia with, 64
  over night sweats, 17
  panic attacks, 13
  as sleep robber, 12–13
  worry, 13, 14
Apnea, sleep. *See* Sleep apnea
Appearance, effect of sleep loss on,
      7–8, 8
Appetite
  control by the hypothalamus, 44
  defined, 45
  hormonal influences on, 22, 25, 44–46,
      49, 168
  increased
    for carbohydrates, 10, 19
    with cortisol, 46, 48, 49, 49
    with neuropeptide Y, 47
    with sleep deprivation, 19, 41, 52
Apples
  recipes
    Apple-Cinnamon Yogurt, 198
    Apples with Honey-Yogurt Dip and
      Candied Walnuts, 196
  spiced apple scent, 163
Apricots
  Brown Rice Pilaf with Apricots and
      Almonds, 223
  Pork Loin Stuffed with Apricots and Wild
      Rice, 202–3
Arcuate nucleus, 44
Aromatherapy, 163–65
Attention deficit/hyperactivity disorder
      (ADHD), 1
Ayurvedic therapies, 121, 126

B

Bamboo sheets, 146
Banana
  bedtime snack, 178
  recipes
    Banana Smoothie, 200
    Frozen Banana Yogurt Pops, 230
Baths, aromatherapy and, 164
Bedroom environment
  air purifiers, 163, 166–67
  air quality, 165–66
  aromatherapy, 163–65
  check of, 133–35
  color, 147, 150–51
  humidity, 163, 165
  lighting, 147–49
    bedside table lamps, 147, <u>150</u>
    blackout curtains, 147, 151–52
    book lights, 147, <u>150</u>
    dimming, 147–48
    natural, 148
    night-lights, 148–49
    overhead fan, 148
    sleep mask use, 147, 151
    from television, 149
  smell, 163–67
  sound in, 152–62
    alarm clocks, 153, 156–58
    earplugs, 153–54
    pet noises, 160
    snoring, 158–59
    sound machines, 153, 154–56
  temperature, 72–73, <u>76</u>
  touch sensation in, 135–46
    comforter, spread, and duvet, 142–43
    mattress, 135–37, <u>137</u>, <u>138</u>
    mattress pads, covers, and protectors, 139
    pillow, **140**, 140–41, **141**
    sheets, 143–46
Bedtime, calculating your, 98–99
Belly fat, 48
Benadryl, <u>172</u>
Beta waves, <u>101</u>, 163
Biological clock. *See* Circadian rhythm
Blackout curtains, 147, 151–52
Black tea
  caffeine in, 110
  before naps, <u>71</u>
Blankets, 75
Bloating, <u>59</u>
Blood alcohol level, 97

Blood pressure
  decrease with
    deep abdominal breathing, 124
    weight loss, 48
  high linked to sleep loss, <u>9</u>, 20
  increase with
    chamomile, <u>181</u>
    snoring, 158
Blood sugar
  increase with sleep loss, 42, 49
  insulin response to, 42
  stabilizing with meals high in protein and
    fiber, <u>169</u>
  vitamin B$_3$ for balancing, 180
Blueberry recipes
  Blueberry Cheesecake Parfaits, 225
  Blueberry-Peanut Butter Shake, 199
Blue light
  effect on circadian rhythm, 15
  light therapy, 120
  melatonin suppression, 69
  night-lights, 149
Body mass index (BMI)
  obesity defined by, 11, 39
  in postmenopausal women, 75
  relationship to sleep quantity, 40, **40**
Body temperature
  bedding influence on, 142
  changes during menstrual cycle, 57
  elevation from exercise, 57, 113, 114
  24-hour rhythm of, 113
Book lights, 147, <u>150</u>
Brain waves, <u>101</u>
Breathing, deep abdominal, 124
Buckwheat
  Buckwheat and Red Lentil Pilaf, 224
B vitamins, <u>59</u>, 180–81

C

Caesarean sections, <u>63</u>
Caffeine
  addiction, steps to curtail, 110–11
  adrenaline increase from, 108
  as anxiety trigger, <u>59</u>
  in black tea, 110
  as diuretic, 111
  dopamine increase from, 108
  eliminating at night, <u>59</u>, 97, 106–11
  energy boost from, 108
  in energy drinks, 108–9
  before naps, <u>71</u>

in soft drinks, 108
withdrawal symptoms, 108
Calcium
calming effect of, 183
food sources, 183
in melatonin production, 171, _179_
for reduction in PMS symptoms, _59_, _65_
vitamin D effect on, 183
Calmness, foods for boosting, 171, _171_
Calories
burned in REM sleep, 41, 43, 112
consumed by teenagers, _25_
decreased burn with sleep loss, 41
decreased consumption with adequate
sleep, 41
empty in alcohol, 112
weight loss and, 23
Cancer
black tea antioxidants for, 110
C-reactive protein as risk marker, 48
estrogen-dependent breast, 185
vitamin D for prevention, 183
Candles, aromatherapy and, 164
Carbohydrates
complex, 171, 173, 176, 178, _179_
eating before bedtime, 176, _179_
effect of growth hormone on utilization of,
50
effect of sleep loss on processing of, 42
glycemic index, 176
increased appetite for
with cortisol, 10, 47
with neuropeptide Y, 47
with poor sleep, 19, 52
serotonin boost from, 171–73, _179_
sleep promotion by, 176
Carbonation, of soda, _169_
Cardiovascular disease. _See_ Heart disease
Cat Stretch with Child's Pose (yoga pose), 122
Chamomile, 165, _181_, _182_
Cheesecake
Blueberry Cheesecake Parfaits, 225
Cherries, tart, 170
Cherry juice, _188_
Chicken recipes
Chicken Breasts with Pine Nuts and
Tangerines, 209
Chicken Pasta Niçoise, 208
Raspberry-Pistachio Crusted Chicken, 210
Children
finding correct bedtime, _161_
Power-Down Hour, 160–62

sleep apnea, _161_
sleep requirements of, _24–25_
survival strategies for kids and sleep,
160–62
Circadian rhythm
blue light effect on, 15
described, 29
differences in personal, 30, _30_
disruption
by evening light exposure, 117–18
metabolic disturbances of, 38
in postpartum moms, 68
exercise effect on, 113
glucose metabolism, 43
malfunctions, 117
PMS effect on, 60–62
progesterone effect on, 60
resetting biological clock, 97
set by
cues of light and darkness, 31, 116–17
melatonin, 31–32
Circulation
decrease with sleep deprivation, 7
increase with yoga postures, 122
Clomiphene (Clomid, Serophene), 70
Clothing, sleep, 75
Coffee
decaffeinated, 111
before naps, _71_
Color, bedroom, 147, 150–51
Combed cotton sheets, 145
Comforter, 142–43
Complexion, effect of sleep loss on, 7–8, _8_
Computer, effect of light from, 14–15
Concentration, decrease with sleep loss, 10
Congestion, nasal, _162_
Continuous positive airway pressure (CPAP)
machine, _17_
Cookies, before bed, 176, 178
Cooking spray, _169_
Copper, food sources of, 184
Corpse Pose (yoga pose), 123
Cortisol
control by feedback loop, 48
decrease with
progressive muscle relaxation (PMR),
124–25
relaxation response, _101_
effect on appetite, 10, 46, 48, 49, _49_
effect on fertility, 70
insomnia and, 70
muscle breakdown by, 46, 47

Cortisol *(cont.)*
  sleep loss effect on, 46, <u>50</u>
  stress and, 46–49, <u>49</u>
Counting backward, 102
CPAP machine, <u>17</u>
Cravings
  cortisol-related, 48
  as PMS symptom, <u>59</u>
  reducing fatigue-induced, 22
C-reactive protein, 48
Curtains, blackout, 147, 151–52

D

Dairy products, 178, <u>179</u>
Daytime sleepiness, in women, 57
DEC2 gene, <u>104</u>
Deep abdominal breathing, 124
Deep sleep, 5, 27–28, 50
Dehydration, by alcohol, 111
Delta sleep, 27–28
Depression
  increase with poor sleep, <u>9</u>, 10
  light therapy for, <u>61</u>
  PMS and, 62
  postpartum, 68–69
  relief with
    foods that boost serotonin, 170
    selective serotonin reuptake inhibitors
     (SSRIs), 172
    seasonal affective disorder (SAD), <u>61</u>,
     118–19
  vitamin B_3 for, 180
Dermatitis, worsening with sleep loss, 8
Dessert recipes
  Blueberry Cheesecake Parfaits, 225
  Frozen Banana Yogurt Pops, 230
  Peachy Frozen Yogurt, 228
  Raspberry Peaches with Greek Yogurt, 229
  Strawberry-Yogurt Shortcakes, 226–27
Diabetes
  C-reactive protein as risk marker, 48
  hyperglycemia, 42
  increase risk with sleep loss, 19–20
  prediabetes, 42
  type 2, <u>8</u>, 12, 19–20, 42
Diet
  key points in *The Sleep Doctor's Diet Plan,*
   <u>169</u>
  sabotage with sleep loss, 52
Diet pills, use of sleeping pills as, <u>32</u>

Diffuser, aromatherapy and, 164
Dimmer switch, 147–48
Diphenhydramine, <u>172</u>
Disordered sleep
  habits contributing to, 36
  sleep disorder distinct from, 33
Diuretic, caffeine as, 111
Dopamine, increase with caffeine, 108
Down, 142
Dreams, 28, 57, 62
Drowsiness
  in PMS, 61–62
  progesterone and, 57, 60, 63, 64
  serotonin and, 171
Duvet, 142–43

E

Early bird, 30, <u>30</u>
Earplugs, 153–54
EEG, 27
Egyptian cotton sheets, 145
Electroencephalograph (EEG), 27
Endorphins, 124
Energy
  boost from caffeine, 108
  saving with blackout curtains, 152
Energy drinks, 108–9, <u>109</u>
Energy expenditure
  components of, 51
  sleep loss effect on, 51–52
Enkephalins, 124
Entrées
  Black Sesame Tofu and Vegetable Stir-Fry,
   218–19
  Chicken Breasts with Pine Nuts and
   Tangerines, 209
  Chicken Pasta Niçoise, 208
  Glazed Halibut with Broccoli and Oranges,
   212–13
  Miso Noodle Bowl, 221
  Pasta Shells with Broccoli, Chickpeas, and
   Tomatoes, 217
  Poached Halibut in Vegetable Broth, 211
  Pork Loin Stuffed with Apricots and Wild
   Rice, 202–3
  Quinoa Stir-Fry with Spinach and Walnuts,
   220
  Raspberry-Pistachio Crusted Chicken, 210
  Roasted Salmon with Mustard-Dill Glaze,
   214

Salmon with Wild Rice Salad, 216
Shrimp Pasta Primavera, 215
Turkey Piccata, 204–5
Turkey Stuffed with Mushrooms and
    Spinach, 206–7
Environment, sleep. *See* Bedroom
    environment
Essential amino acid, 170
Essential oils, 165
Estradiol, 72
Estrogen
    increase during rapid eye movement (REM)
        sleep, 57
    isoflavones, estrogen-like effects of, 73
    in menopause, 73
    during menstrual cycle, 60
    phytoestrogens, 185
Exercise
    avoidance before bed, 59, 97, 112–15, 116
    benefits of, 112–13
    finding "perfect" time for, 115
    list of activities, 116
    in morning sunlight, 59, 67–68
    thermogenic hypothesis, 114
    while traveling, 127
    yoga, 121–23
Exercise journal, 115
Eyes, effect of sleep loss on appearance,
    7, 8
Eyeshade (eye mask), 147, 151

F

Fat
    abdominal (belly, visceral), 48
    effect of growth hormone on utilization of,
        50
    food stored as, 43
    hormonal influences on storage
        cortisol, 46
        insulin, 49
    loss with adequate sleep, 41
    neck, 74
Fatigue
    in PMS, 61–62
    progesterone and, 57, 60
Ferritin, level in restless legs syndrome, 35
Fertility, 69–70
Fiber
    blood sugar stabilization and, 169
    sources of, 179

Fibromyalgia, 175
Fight or flight response, 7, 101
Filter
    air, 163, 166–67
    for television or computer light, 149
Fish recipes
    Glazed Halibut with Broccoli and Oranges,
        212–13
    Poached Halibut in Vegetable Broth, 211
    Roasted Salmon with Mustard-Dill Glaze,
        214
    Salmon with Wild Rice Salad, 216
5-HTP, 182
Flame-retardant bedding, 143
Focus, inability with poor sleep, 7, 8, 10
Folic acid, 181
Follicle-stimulating hormone, 60
Follicular phase, of menstrual cycle, 58, 60
Food. *See also* Recipes; *specific foods and
        food groups*
    glycemic index, 176
    myths and facts, 175–76, 178
    portion control, 174
    sleep busters, 179
    sleep-inducing, 170–73
    snacks, 173–74
    soy, 185, 188
    spices, 177
    thermic effect of, 51
    vitamins and minerals, 180–85
Fragrance, 163–65

G

Garlic, 177
Gastroesophageal reflux disease (GERD), 63
Ghrelin
    effect of poor sleep on, 45–46, 49, 50
    effect of stress on, 49
    effect on energy expenditure, 51
    secretion by the stomach, 45
    in teenagers, 25
Glamour Sleep Challenge, 21–23
Glucose metabolism, 42–43, 43
Glucose tolerance, 39
Glycemic index, 176
Growth hormone
    reduced with sleep loss, 50, 50
    secretion during deep-sleep stage, 5, 27,
        50
Guided imagery, 125–26

H

Hair, effect of sleep loss on, 7, <u>8</u>
Halibut recipes
   Glazed Halibut with Broccoli and Oranges,
      212–13
   Poached Halibut in Vegetable Broth, 211
Healing, during deep sleep, 27–28
Heartburn, 63, 64
Heart disease
   C-reactive protein as risk marker, 48
   link to sleep loss, <u>9</u>, 20
HEPA filter, 166–67
Herbal tea, <u>177</u>
Herbs, <u>177</u>, <u>182</u>
High-efficiency particulate air (HEPA) filter,
   166–67
Homeostasis, 42
Hormones
   appetite, 22, <u>25</u>, 44–45
   cortisol
      control by feedback loop, 48
      decrease with progressive muscle
         relaxation (PMR), 124–25
      decrease with relaxation response, <u>101</u>
      effect on appetite, 10, 46, 48, 49, <u>49</u>
      effect on fertility, 70
      insomnia and, 70
      muscle breakdown by, 46, 47
      sleep loss effect on, 46, <u>50</u>
      stress and, 46–49, <u>49</u>
   follicle-stimulating hormone, 60
   functions of, 44
   ghrelin
      appetite and, 22, <u>25</u>, 44–46, <u>49</u>, <u>50</u>, 168
      effect of poor sleep on, 45–46, <u>49</u>, 50
      effect of stress on, <u>49</u>
      effect on energy expenditure, 51
      secretion by the stomach, 45
      in teenagers, <u>25</u>
   growth hormone, 5, 27, 50, <u>50</u>
   insulin
      effect of sleep loss on production, 7, 43
      glucose metabolism and, 42, 49
      tryptophan promotion by, 176, <u>179</u>
      vitamin D effect on function, 183
   leptin
      appetite and, 22, <u>25</u>, 44–45, <u>49</u>, <u>50</u>
      decreased production with low vitamin
         D level, 118
      effect of poor sleep on, 45, <u>49</u>, 50
      effect of stress on, <u>49</u>

infertility and, 70
influence on perception of sweetness,
   52
receptors in obese individuals, 45
in teenagers, <u>25</u>
vitamin D importance for production of,
   <u>59</u>
light therapy and, <u>61</u>
during menopause, 73
sleep disruption in women and, 57–58
Hot flashes, 71, 72, 73
Hot-water bottle, to warm feet, 75
Humidity, 163, 165
Hummus
   Roasted Pepper Hummus, 194
Hunger. *See also* Appetite
   decrease with adequate sleep, 168–69
   defined, 45
   hormonal control of, 44–46, <u>49</u>, <u>50</u>
   during menstrual cycle, 60
5-hydroxytryptophan, <u>182</u>
Hyperglycemia, 42
Hypoallergenic bedding, 143
Hypoglycemia, 42
Hypothalamus, 15, 44, 48

I

Immune system, weakened with sleep loss, <u>9</u>,
   10–11
Infertility, 69–70
Inflammation
   C-reactive protein as proinflammatory
      marker, 48
   with gastroesophageal reflux disease
      (GERD), 63
Inflammation, increase with sleep loss, 19
Insomnia
   causes
      anxiety, 64
      folic acid deficiency, 181
      zinc deficiency, 184
   during menstrual cycle, 60
   perimenopausal, 70–72
   postmenopausal, 76
   postpartum, 68
   during pregnancy, 64
   as secondary sleep disorder, 33, 34
   treatment
      acupuncture, <u>121</u>
      light therapy, 118
      tryptophan supplements, 175–76

Insulin
  effect of sleep loss on production, 7, 43
  glucose metabolism and, 42, 49
  tryptophan promotion by, 176, _179_
  vitamin D effect on function, 183
Insulin resistance, 19, 20, 49
Internet, as sleep robber, 14–15
Iron
  deficiency and restless legs syndrome, 184,
    _184_
  food sources of, 184
Isoflavones, 73, 185

J

Jasmine scent, 163
Jersey sheets, 145
Jet lag, 60
Juice
  eliminating from diet, _169_
  tart cherry, _188_

K

Kava, _182_

L

Lamp, bedside table, 148, _150_
Lavender
  aromatherapy, 163–64, 165
  massage oil, 129
  supplement, _182_
LDL cholesterol levels, decrease with weight
    loss, 48
Lean body mass, loss of, 41
Leg cramps, _66_
Lemon scent, 163
Leptin
  appetite and, 22, _25_, 44–45, _49_, _50_
  effect of poor sleep on, 45, _49_, 50
  effect of stress on, _49_
  infertility and, 70
  influence on perception of sweetness, 52
  receptors in obese individuals, 45
  in teenagers, _25_
  vitamin D importance for production of,
    _59_, 118
Light therapy, _61_, 118, 120
Lignins, 185
Limbic system, 163
Linen sheets, 145

Liquids, increased intake to reduce sodium,
    _59_
Luteal phase, of menstrual cycle, 57, 58, 60

M

Magnesium
  food sources of, 184
  mood enhancement from, _59_
  as muscle relaxant, _59_
  in serotonin production, 171
  supplements, 183
Mango
  Mango-Soy Smoothie, 201
Massage, self, 128–29
Massage oil, 129, 164
Mattress
  average lifespan of, 135
  health effects of improper, _137_
  Life Cycle™ chart, _138_
  pads, covers, and protectors, 139
  when to buy a new mattress, 135–37
Mattress pads, 139
Mattress protector, 139
Meals. _See also_ Recipes
  number and frequency of, _169_
  sleep-friendly examples, 173
Meditation, 126–28
Melatonin
  blue light suppression of, 69
  in cherries, 170, _188_
  circadian rhythm set by, 31–32
  decrease production in luteal phase of
    menstrual cycle, 57
  disruption from bedroom lighting, 147,
    148, 149, 151
  dosage, _187_
  effect of computer monitor light on release,
    15
  functions of, _186_
  during PMS, 61
  secretion from pineal gland, 15, 31, 32, 68,
    119, _186_
  sunlight and regulation of, 15, _59_, _109_, 116
  supplements, 31–32, _186–87_
  tryptophan as building block for, 170, _179_
Memory
  consolidation of, 7
  poor with sleep loss, _8_, 10
Menopause
  hormones during, 73
  sleep tips for, 72–73, 75

Menopause *(cont.)*
  symptoms, 73
  weight gain after, 74
Menstrual cycle
  body temperature changes during, 57
  hormonal changes during, 57, 60
  melatonin production during, 57
  phases, 58, 60
  PMS, 60–62, <u>61</u>
Menstruation, 60
Metabolic disturbances, from lack of sleep,
    20
Metabolic rate
  decrease with inadequate sleep, 6, 38
  resting, 51
Metabolic syndrome, 12, 20
Metabolism
  alcohol, 112
  boost from exercise, 112
  energy expenditure, 51–52
  glucose, 42–43, **43**
  during menstrual cycle, 60
Milk, warm before bed, 178
Minerals, 183–85
Mineral water, <u>169</u>
Monitor, effect of light from computer,
    14–15
Moodiness
  from circadian rhythm disruption, 117
  increase with poor sleep, <u>9</u>, 10
  link to low vitamin D level, 118
Morning light. *See* Sunlight
Motion-sensor night-lights, 149
Multitasking, by women, <u>14</u>
Muscle breakdown by cortisol, 46, 47
Muscle relaxant, magnesium as, <u>59</u>
Muscle relaxation, progressive, 124–25
Mushroom recipes
  Roasted Squash and Shiitakes, 222
  Turkey Stuffed with Mushrooms and
    Spinach, 206–7
Music, relaxation effects of, 129–31, <u>130</u>
Muslin sheets, 145

N

Naps
  Nap-a-Latte, <u>71</u>
  in pregnancy, <u>66</u>
  tips for great afternoon nap, <u>69</u>
Nasal congestion, <u>162</u>

Neti pots, <u>162</u>
Neural tube defects, 181
Neuropeptide Y, 47
Niacin (vitamin B$_3$), 180
Night-lights, <u>66</u>, 148–49
Nightmares, 64, 112
Night owl, 30, <u>30</u>
Night sweats, 16–17, 71, 73, 185
Nighttime awakenings, 68, 73, 181
Nighttime Goddess Stretch (yoga pose), 123
Noise
  reducing with
    curtains, 152
    earplugs, 153–54
  white noise machines, 153, 154–56
Non-rapid eye movement (NREM) sleep, 27,
    28, 112
NREM sleep, 27, **28**, 112
Nutmeg, <u>177</u>

O

Obesity
  C-reactive protein as risk marker, 48
  defined by body mass index, 11, 39
  with sleep loss, 5, <u>8</u>, 11–12, <u>11</u>18–19,
    39–40
  vitamin D unavailability, 118
Olfactory nerve, 163
Olive oil cooking spray, <u>169</u>
Oranges
  Glazed Halibut with Broccoli and Oranges,
    212–13
Osteoporosis, 183
Overhead fan lighting, 148–49
Overtime, and sleep quantity decline, 12
Overweight, as determined by body mass
    index (BMI), 39
Ovulation, 57, 58, 60, 70

P

Pain sensitivity, increase with poor sleep, <u>8</u>,
    9–10
Panic attacks, 13
Pasta recipes
  Chicken Pasta Niçoise, 208
  Miso Noodle Bowl, 221
  Pasta Shells with Broccoli, Chickpeas, and
    Tomatoes, 217
  Shrimp Pasta Primavera, 215

Peaches
   Peachy Frozen Yogurt, 228
   Raspberry Peaches with Greek Yogurt, 229
Peanut butter
   in bedtime snacks, <u>179</u>, 199
   Blueberry-Peanut Butter Shake, 199
Percale sheets, 145, 146
Perimenopause, 70–72, 73
Periodic limb movements in sleep, 35
Pets, noisy, 160
Phosphorus, vitamin D effect on, 183
Phytoestrogens, 185
Pic-a-pillow chart, **141**
Pillow, **140**, 140–41, **141**
Pillow sachet, 164
Pillow spray, 164
Pima cotton sheets, 145
Pineal gland
   light influence on, <u>61</u>, 68, <u>109</u>, 119
   melatonin production by, 15, 31, 32, 68,
      119, <u>186</u>
Pituitary gland, 60, <u>61</u>
Placebo, <u>172</u>
Plain weave sheets, 146
Plug-ins, aromatherapy and, 164
PMDD, 62
PMR, 124–25
PMS
   biological clock affected by, 60–62
   light therapy for, <u>61</u>
   premenstrual dysphoric disorder (PMDD), 62
   sleep tips for, <u>59</u>
Pocket depth, sheet, 144
Polyester, 142, 146
Pork recipes
   Pork Loin Stuffed with Apricots and Wild
      Rice, 202–3
Portion control, 174
Postmenopausal sleep disorders, 75–77
Postpartum sleeplessness, 64–69, <u>65</u>
Power-Down Hour, 105–6, 160–62
Pranayama, 122
Prefrontal cortex, 7
Pregnancy
   Caesarean sections, <u>63</u>
   first trimester, 64, <u>66</u>
   gastroesophageal reflux disease (GERD)
      during, 63
   labor length, <u>63</u>
   postpartum sleeplessness, 64–65, <u>65</u>,
      67–69

second trimester, 64, <u>66</u>
   sleep tips for, <u>66</u>
   sleep variations during, 63–64
   third trimester, 64, <u>66</u>
Premenstrual dysphoric disorder (PMDD), 62
Progesterone
   fatigue and drowsiness from, 57, 60, 63, 64
   in menopause, 73
   during menstrual cycle, 57, 60
   in pregnancy, 63, 64
Progressive muscle relaxation (PMR),
      124–25
Proinflammatory markers, 48
Protein
   blood sugar stabilization and, <u>169</u>
   sleep interference by high-protein meals,
      176, <u>179</u>
   in snacks, 174, 176

Q

Quality of sleep
   factors affecting, 32
   music, benefits of, 129–30
   recording in sleep diary, 86–93
   sleep apnea and, <u>17</u>
Quantity of sleep
   calculating your needed amount, 99
   effect of overtime work on, 12
   recording in sleep diary, 86–93
   relationship to body mass index (BMI), 40,
      40
   required in children, <u>24–25</u>
   signs of insufficient, 33
   United States average amount in adults, 11
Quinoa
   Quinoa Stir-Fry with Spinach and Walnuts,
      220
Quiz, sleep disruption, <u>84–85</u>

R

Rapid eye movement (REM) sleep
   calories burned in, 6, 41, 43, 112
   described, 28, 28–29
   dreams, 28
   estrogen increase during, 57
   lengthened by vitamin B$_3$, 180
   during menstrual cycle, 60
   as mental restoration stage of sleep, 28
   reduced by alcohol, 112

Raspberry
  Raspberry Peaches with Greek Yogurt, 229
  Raspberry-Pistachio Crusted Chicken, 210
Recipes
  calming foods and nutrients in, 191
  desserts
    Blueberry Cheesecake Parfaits, 225
    Frozen Banana Yogurt Pops, 230
    Peachy Frozen Yogurt, 228
    Raspberry Peaches with Greek Yogurt, 229
    Strawberry-Yogurt Shortcakes, 226–27
  entrées
    Black Sesame Tofu and Vegetable
      Stir-Fry, 218–19
    Chicken Breasts with Pine Nuts and
      Tangerines, 209
    Chicken Pasta Niçoise, 208
    Glazed Halibut with Broccoli and
      Oranges, 212–13
    Miso Noodle Bowl, 221
    Pasta Shells with Broccoli, Chickpeas,
      and Tomatoes, 217
    Poached Halibut in Vegetable Broth, 211
    Pork Loin Stuffed with Apricots and
      Wild Rice, 202–3
    Quinoa Stir-Fry with Spinach and
      Walnuts, 220
    Raspberry-Pistachio Crusted Chicken,
      210
    Roasted Salmon with Mustard-Dill
      Glaze, 214
    Salmon with Wild Rice Salad, 216
    Shrimp Pasta Primavera, 215
    Turkey Piccata, 204–5
    Turkey Stuffed with Mushrooms and
      Spinach, 206–7
  sides
    Brown Rice Pilaf with Apricots and
      Almonds, 223
    Buckwheat and Red Lentil Pilaf, 224
    Roasted Squash and Shiitakes, 222
  snacks
    Apple-Cinnamon Yogurt, 198
    Apples with Honey-Yogurt Dip and
      Candied Walnuts, 196
    Banana Smoothie, 200
    Blueberry-Peanut Butter Shake, 199
    Cheese and Crackers, 197
    Mango-Soy Smoothie, 201
    Parmesan Cheese Toasts, 193

    Roasted Lemon-Herb Tofu, 195
    Roasted Pepper Hummus, 194
Red wine, antioxidants in, 112
Relaxation methods
  aromatherapy, 163–65
  deep abdominal breathing, 124
  meditation, 126–28
  music, 129–31
  progressive muscle relaxation (PMR), 124–25
  self-massage, 128–29
  visualization, 125–26
Relaxation response, 101, 126
REM sleep. See Rapid eye movement (REM)
  sleep
Restless legs syndrome, 33–34, 35, 60, 184,
  184
Rice recipes
  Brown Rice Pilaf with Apricots and
    Almonds, 223
  Pork Loin Stuffed with Apricots and Wild
    Rice, 202–3
  Salmon with Wild Rice Salad, 216
RLS. See Restless legs syndrome
Rock-a-Bye Roll (yoga pose), 123
Room color, 147, 150–51
Room lighting, 147–49
Rosacea, worsening with sleep loss, 8
Rules for better sleep, 96–131
  alcohol avoidance before bedtime, 97, 111–12
  caffeine elimination after 2:00 PM, 97,
    106–11
  exercise avoidance before bed, 97, 112–15,
    116
  morning sunlight, 97, 116–20
  stick to one sleep schedule, 97, 98–106

S

SAD, 61, 118–19
Saline solution, 162
Salmon recipes
  Roasted Salmon with Mustard-Dill Glaze,
    214
  Salmon with Wild Rice Salad, 216
Sateen sheets, 146
Satin sheets, 146
Scents, 163–65
Sciatic nerve pain, 64
Seasonal affective disorder (SAD), 61, 118–19
Selective serotonin reuptake inhibitors
  (SSRIs), 172

Self-massage, 128–29
Senses
    sight, 146–52
    smell, 163–67
    sound, 152–62
    touch, 135–46
Sensitive sleepers, 82–83, 85
Serophene (clomiphene), 70
Serotonin
    boost from
        foods, 7, 10, 170–73, _171_, _179_
        light therapy, _61_
        magnesium, _59_
        self-massage, 128
        vitamin B₆, _59_, 180
    pain sensitivity increase with decrease in,
        8, 9
    seasonal affective disorder (SAD) and, 119
    selective serotonin reuptake inhibitors
        (SSRIs), 172
    sleep loss effect on, 9, _49_
    stress effect on, _49_
    tryptophan as building block for, 58, 170,
        175
Shakes
    Blueberry-Peanut Butter Shake, 199
Sheets, selecting
    feel, 144–46
    fit, 144
    importance of, 143
    size, 144
    thread count, 145
    types, 145–46
Shift workers, 117
Short sleepers, _104_
Shrimp
    Shrimp Pasta Primavera, 215
Side dish recipes
    Brown Rice Pilaf with Apricots and
        Almonds, 223
    Buckwheat and Red Lentil Pilaf, 224
    Roasted Squash and Shiitakes, 222
Silk bedding, 143, 146
Sinus wash, _162_
Skin, effect of sleep loss on, 7–8, _8_
Sleep
    as sensory experience, 133
    United States average amount in adults, 11
Sleep apnea
    alcohol consumption and, 97
    in children, _161_

description of, 34
in postmenopausal women, 77
signs and symptoms of, _35_
snoring and, _17_, 158–59
treatment, _17_
Sleep cycle
    length, 29, 99
    number of cycles required, 29
    stages of sleep, 27–29
Sleep debt
    calculating, 99–100
    defined, 54
    repaying, 99, 169
Sleep deprivation. _See_ Sleep loss
Sleep diary
    described, 81–82
    examples of patient use, 55, 107
    forms
        week 1, 86–87
        week 2, 88–89
        week 3, 90–91
        week 4, 92–93
Sleep disorders
    consequences of untreated, 34
    described, 33–34
    insomnia
        from anxiety, 64
        light therapy for, 118
        during menstrual cycle, 60
        perimenopausal, 70–72
        in postmenopausal women, 76
        postpartum, 68
        during pregnancy, 64
        as secondary sleep disorder, 33, 34
    periodic limb movements in sleep, 35
    postmenopausal, 75–77
    primary, 33
    restless legs syndrome, 33–34, 35, 60, 184,
        _184_
    secondary, 33
    sleep apnea as, 34, _35_
Sleep disruption quiz, _84–85_
Sleep drive, 29
Sleep environment. _See_ Bedroom
    environment
Sleep hygiene
    identified with sleep diary, 82
    importance of, 82–83
    leading to disordered sleep, 36
    rules for better sleep, 96–131
Sleeping pills, _32_

Sleep loss
  causes
    anxiety, 12–13, _14_
    blue light, 15
    Internet addiction, 14–15
    sleep apnea, _17_
  effects of, 6–12, _8–9_, 18–20
    on appetite hormone levels, 45–46, _50_
    on cortisol secretion, 48, 49
    on energy expenditure, 51–52
    focus and memory problems, 7, _8_, 10
    on growth hormone, 50, _50_
    on hair, 7, _8_
    heart disease, _9_, 20
    high blood pressure, _9_, 20
    on hormones, _49_, _50_
    immune system impairment, _9_, 10–11
    metabolic disturbances, 20
    moodiness and depression, _9_, 10
    pain sensitivity increase, _8_, 9–10
    on skin, 7–8, _8_
    type 2 diabetes, _8_, 12, 19–20
    weight gain, _8_, _11_, 11–12, 18–19, 39–41
Sleep mask, 147, 151
Sleep mood, 133
Sleep pacemaker. _See_ Circadian rhythm
Sleep sanctuary, 132, 135
Sleep schedule
  calculating sleep debt, 99–100
  family history of short sleepers, _104_
  figuring out your bedtime, 98–99
  Power-Down Hour, 105–6
  sleep amount required, 99
  sleep window, 100
  sticking to one, 97, 98–106
  stress-tackling tips for weight loss, 100–102
  Worry Journal, 103, 105
Sleep-wake schedule
  conflicts with, _30_
  regulating naturally, _187_
Sleepwear, 75
Sleep window, 100
Smell, sensation in bedroom environment, 163–67
Smoothies
  Banana Smoothie, 200
  Mango-Soy Smoothie, 201
Snacks
  examples, 174
  increase consumption with poor sleep, 19, 50–51

nighttime, 21, 173–74, 176, 178, _179_
protein in, 174, 176
recipes
  Apple-Cinnamon Yogurt, 198
  Apples with Honey-Yogurt Dip and Candied Walnuts, 196
  Banana Smoothie, 200
  Blueberry-Peanut Butter Shake, 199
  Cheese and Crackers, 197
  Mango-Soy Smoothie, 201
  Parmesan Cheese Toasts, 193
  Roasted Lemon-Herb Tofu, 195
  Roasted Pepper Hummus, 194
sleeping instead of snacking, 21
Snoring
  coping with sounds of, 158–59
  incidence of, 158
  sleep apnea and, _35_, 158–59
Sodas, eliminating from diet, _169_
Sodium, link to water retention and bloating, _59_
Sound
  alarm clocks, 153, 156–58
  machines, 153, 154–56
  reducing with
    curtains, 152
    earplugs, 153–54
  sleep disrupting, 152–53
    children, 160–62
    pet noise, 160
    snoring, 158–59
Sound machines, 153, 154–56
Sound masking, 155
Soy
  foods, 185, 188
  hot flashes decrease with, 73
  phytoestrogens in, 185
Soybeans, 185
Speakers, sound machine, 155
Sphincter, 63
Spinach
  Quinoa Stir-Fry with Spinach and Walnuts, 220
  Turkey Stuffed with Mushrooms and Spinach, 206–7
Spread, bed, 142–43
Squash
  Roasted Squash and Shiitakes, 222
SSRIs, 172
Stages of sleep
  cycling through, 29
  mental restorative, 28

non-rapid eye movement (NREM)
  stage 1 sleep, 27, **28**
  stage 2 sleep, 27, **28**
  stage 3 and 4 sleep (deep sleep/delta
    sleep), 27–28, **28**
  physical restorative, 28
  rapid eye movement (REM), 6, **28**, 28–29
Stir fry recipes
  Black Sesame Tofu and Vegetable Stir-Fry,
    218–19
  Quinoa Stir-Fry with Spinach and Walnuts,
    220
Strawberry
  Strawberry-Yogurt Shortcakes, 226–27
Stress
  chronic, 47–48
  cortisol production and, 46–49, _49_
  fight or flight response, _101_
  increased vitamin and mineral needs with,
    180
  infertility and, 70
  reduction with
    deep abdominal breathing, 124
    exercise, 113
    meditation, 126–28
    progressive muscle relaxation (PMR),
      124–25
    self-massage, 128–29
    visualization, 125–26
    yoga, 122
  stress-tackling tips for weight loss,
    100–102
  weight gain with, 48–49
  in working mothers, 101–2
  Worry Journal, 103, 105
Stretching, 115
Sugar pills, _172_
Sunlight
  blue light in, 15
  exercising in morning, _59_, 67–68
  increasing your amount of, 119–20
  melatonin regulation and, 15, _59_, _109_, 116
  seasonal affective disorder (SAD), _61_,
    118–19
  vitamin D and, _59_, 181, 183
Supplements
  calcium, 183
  effect on cortisol, 46
  "fat-burning," 46
  iron, _184_
  melatonin, 31–32, _186–87_
  natural, _182_

tryptophan, 175–76, _182_
vitamin D, 119, 183
Sweetness, perception of, 52

T

Tangerines
  Chicken Breasts with Pine Nuts and
    Tangerines, 209
Tart cherry juice, _188_
Teenagers, sleep deprivation in, _25_
Television, light from, 149
Temperature
  bedroom, 72–73, _76_
  finding optimal sleep, 74–75
Tension, reduction of
  with meditation, 126–28
  with progressive muscle relaxation, 125–26
  with self-massage, 128–29
  with visualization, 125–26
  with yoga, 121–23
Thermic effect of food, 51
Thermogenic hypothesis, 114
Thread count, sheet, 145
Tofu
  preparation tips, _195_
  recipes
    Black Sesame Tofu and Vegetable
      Stir-Fry, 218–19
    Roasted Lemon-Herb Tofu, 195
Touch, sensation in bedroom environment,
    135–46
Touch dimmer, 148
Touch therapy, 128–29
Travel, sleep disruptions during, _127_
Triglyceride levels, decrease with weight loss,
    48
Tryptophan
  as essential amino acid, 170
  food sources of, 171
  5-hydroxytryptophan, _182_
  as serotonin building block, 58, 170, 175
  supplements, 175–76, _182_
  in turkey, 175
  vitamin B$_3$ for increased effectiveness of, 180
TUMS, _59_
Turkey
  recipes
    Turkey Piccata, 204–5
    Turkey Stuffed with Mushrooms and
      Spinach, 206–7
  tryptophan in, 175

Turmeric, <u>177</u>
Tyrosine, 176, <u>179</u>

V

Valerian, <u>182</u>
Visceral fat, 48
Visualization, 125–26
Vitamin B₃ (niacin), 180
Vitamin B₆, serotonin boost from, <u>59</u>, 180
Vitamin B₁₂, 181
Vitamin D, <u>59</u>, 118–19, 181, 183
Vivid dreams, 57, 62

W

Walnut recipes
  Apples with Honey-Yogurt Dip and
    Candied Walnuts, 196
  Buckwheat and Red Lentil Pilaf, 224
  Quinoa Stir-Fry with Spinach and Walnuts,
    220
Water, flavored, <u>169</u>
Water retention, <u>59</u>
Weight gain
  after menopause, 74
  causes in women, 4
  hormonal influences, 45–51
    cortisol, 46–49, <u>49</u>, <u>50</u>
    growth hormone, <u>49</u>, 50, <u>50</u>
    leptin and ghrelin, 44–46, <u>50</u>
  with inadequate sleep, 6, 11–12, 18–19, 38–53
  in postpartum moms, 65
Weight loss
  decrease in proinflammatory markers with,
    48
  with increased sleep, 22
  key points in *The Sleep Doctor's Diet Plan*,
    <u>169</u>
  stress-tackling tips for, 100–102
White noise machines, 153, 154–56
Whole grains, <u>179</u>
Wine, antioxidants in, 112
Women, unique sleep challenges of
  hormone-related, 57–58
  menopause, 72–74, 75

menstrual cycle and, 58–62, 59, 61
  perimenopausal insomnia, 70–72
  postmenopausal sleep disorders,
    75–77
  postpartum, 64–69, <u>65</u>
  pregnancy, 62–64, <u>63</u>, <u>66</u>
Wool, 142
Worry, 13, <u>14</u>
Worry Journal, 103, 105
Wrinkles, increase with sleep loss,
  7–8, <u>8</u>

Y

Ylang-ylang, 165
Yoga
  hatha, 121–22
  poses
    Cat Stretch with Child's Pose, 122
    Corpse Pose, 123
    Nighttime Goddess Stretch, 123
    Rock-a-Bye Roll, 123
  pranayama, 122
  tension relief with, 121–23
Yogurt
  in bedtime snacks, <u>179</u>
  dessert recipes
    Frozen Banana Yogurt Pops, 230
    Peachy Frozen Yogurt, 228
    Raspberry Peaches with Greek Yogurt,
      229
    Strawberry-Yogurt Shortcakes,
      226–27
  smoothie recipes
    Banana Smoothie, 200
    Mango-Soy Smoothie, 201
  snack recipes
    Apple-Cinnamon Yogurt, 198
    Apples with Honey-Yogurt Dip and
      Candied Walnuts, 196

Z

Zinc
  deficiency and insomnia, 184
  food sources of, 184